Diet/Health

D0470578

newbody

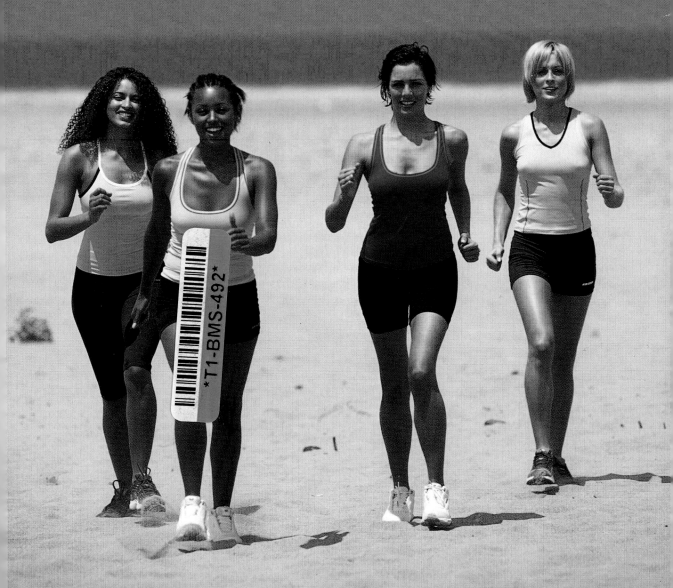

T1-BMS-492

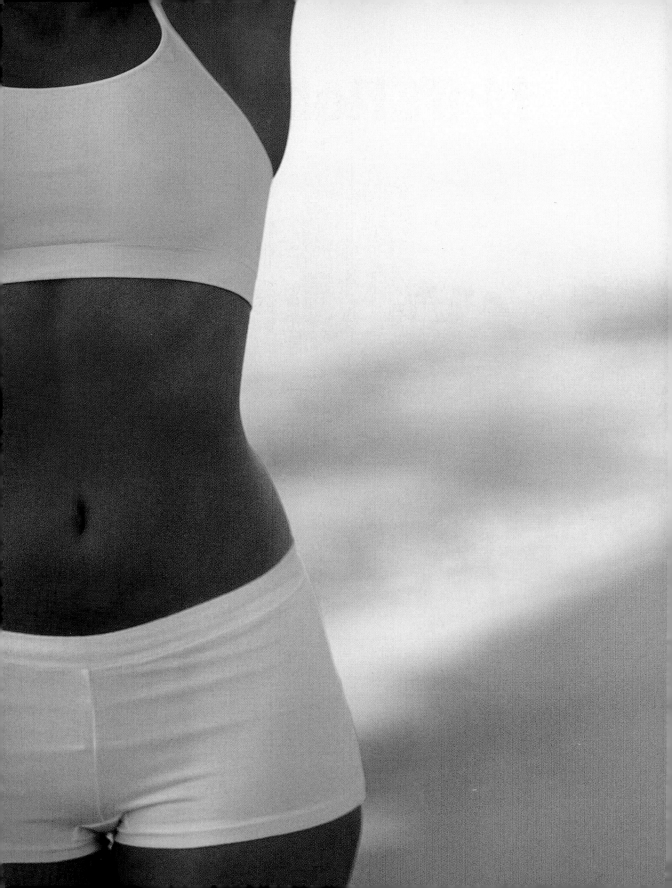

Matt Roberts

newbody

LONDON, NEW YORK, MELBOURNE, MUNICH and DELHI

Project Editor Charmaine Yabsley
Art Direction and Design XAB Design
Managing Editor Gillian Roberts
Managing Art Editor Karen Sawyer
Category Publisher Mary-Clare Jerram
Art Director Carole Ash
DTP Designer Sonia Charbonnier
Production Controller Joanna Bull
Photographer Russell Sadur
Photographer's Assistant Nina Duncan

First American Edition, 2003

Published in the United States by
DK Publishing, Inc.
375 Hudson Street
New York, New York 10014

03 04 05 06 07 10 9 8 7 6 5 4 3 2 1

Copyright © 2003 Dorling Kindersley Limited
Text copyright © 2003 Matt Roberts Personal Training

Always consult your doctor before starting a fitness and/or
nutrition program if you have any health concerns.

All rights reserved under International and Pan-American
Copyright Conventions. No part of this publication may
be reproduced, stored in a retrieval system, or transmitted
in any form or by any means, electronic, mechanical,
photocopying, recording or otherwise, without the prior
written permission of the copyright owner. Published in
Great Britain by Dorling Kindersley Limited.

A Cataloging-in-Publication record for this book
is available from the Library of Congress.

ISBN 0-7894-9937-1

Color reproduced by Colourscan, Singapore
Printed and bound in Germany by MOHN Media and
Mohndruck GmbH

Discover more at
www.dk.com

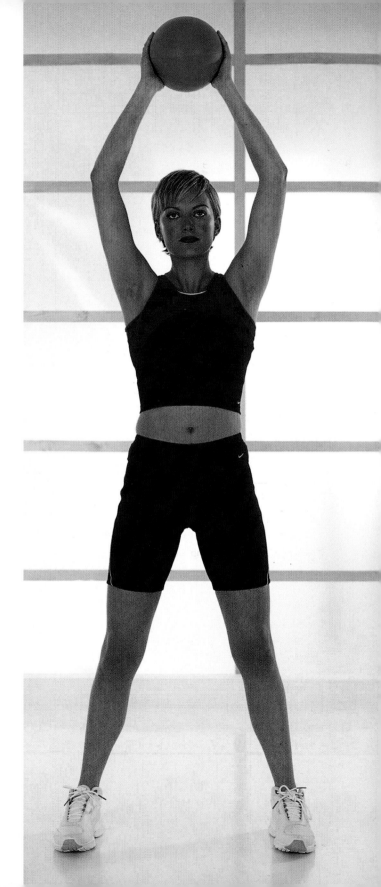

contents

about the book

One of the most common questions or requests I hear from clients, friends, and family is, "How can I change my body shape?" It seems no matter what our individual attributes of hair color, skin tone, or stature, we want the opposite of what we have. Of course it's healthy to accept yourself as you are, but it's reassuring, too, to know that you can change certain aspects. If you dislike the color of your hair, you can dye it. If pale skin makes you unhappy, get a fake tan, or use makeup. There's not much to be done if you fret about your height, but I can certainly help you achieve your ideal body shape.

The first step in reaching that goal is to accept the underlying shape you were born with. You are what you are. The secret to changing your body shape is to make the most of the one you have (I'll show you how), and learn a few tricks along the way.

It's important to grasp the concept that there is no such thing as a "perfect" body shape. Many women envy the straight-up-and-down tube shape, or the well-proportioned curves of the hourglass. But every shape has positive and negative aspects. The tube, though relatively shapeless, looks the best in clothes; the hourglass, with its voluptuous curves, is possibly the sexiest shape; the pear has elegant arms and a handsome back, perfect features in that little black dress; the apple boasts the best legs of them all.

In the past, if you had large hips, you were probably encouraged to spend hours trying to "reduce" that area—undoubtedly with little success. Instead of trying to diminish "problem" areas, we are going to create the most well-proportioned figure for your shape by doing exercises to balance your top with your bottom, and your front with your back.

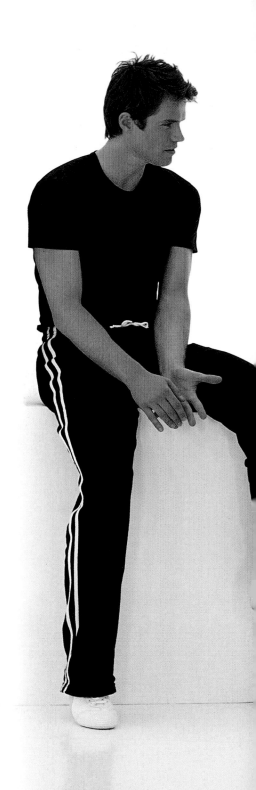

By developing good muscle tone, reducing body fat, and improving your posture, you'll look stronger, leaner, and taller. Although this is not a diet book, it's more than likely that you will lose fat as a bonus of your training program, and your clothes should fit better. To make the most of your great new figure, take a look at the "what to wear" feature for each body shape. Knowing what suits you and what to avoid is the perfect adjunct to your new body.

Know your shape on pages 8–9 will help you to identify yours. Once you have, turn to the relevant pages for your shape to read more about it, your workout goals, and tips for eating well. Then make a commitment to do the workouts that are specifically designed for your shape: they're easily identified by the appropriate symbol. Stick with your commitment, and I promise that you'll be rewarded with a fitter body in the best possible shape.

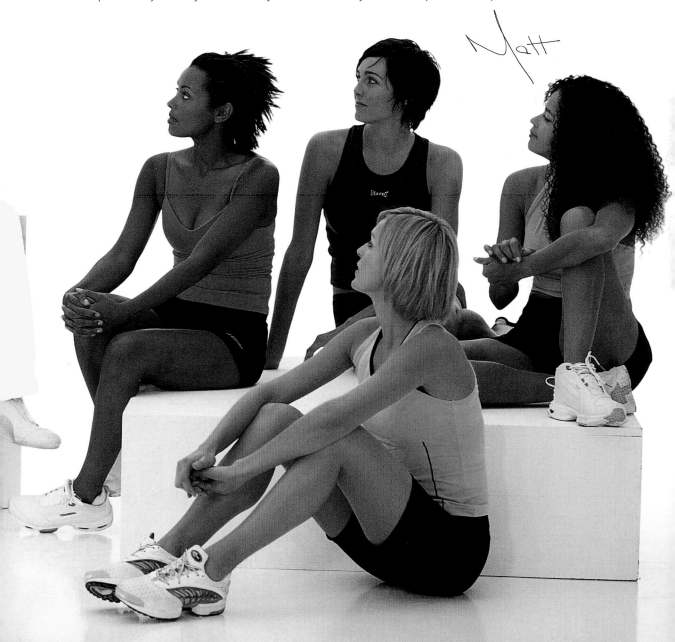

know your shape

Although genes determine your natural body shape, other factors such as diet, lifestyle, and exercise play an important role in helping you make the best of your personal attributes.

The workouts I have designed for this book show you how to capitalize on your natural assets, but before starting the exercise programs, identify which of the four body shapes is yours.

You have a tube body shape if

- your bust, waist, and hips are a similar width
- you have an undefined waist
- your figure is basically straight up and down

If this sounds like you, turn to your detailed body profile on pages 10–15.

You have an apple body shape if

- you have a full bust, waist, and upper back
- you tend to hold weight around your abdomen
- your rear end is small and flat

If this sounds like you, turn to your detailed body profile on pages 16–21.

You have an hourglass body shape if

- your shoulders and hips are a similar width
- you have a well-defined waist
- your figure has the classic female curves

If this sounds like you, turn to your detailed body profile on pages 22–27.

You have a pear body shape if

- your hips are wider than your shoulders and bust
- you have a well-defined waist and shapely, prominent backside

If this sounds like you, turn to your detailed body profile on pages 28–33.

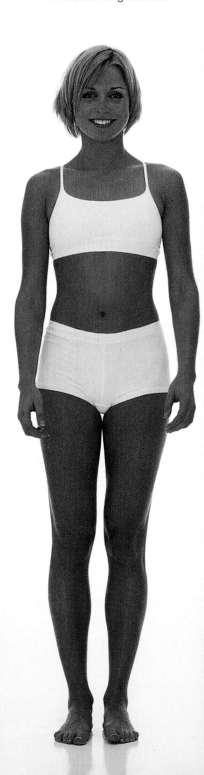

tube
shoulders, waist, and hips are a similar width; limbs are long and lean

apple

shoulders are broad,
rear end is small and flat;
appearance is top-heavy

hourglass

shoulders and hips
are a similar width;
waist is small and curved

pear

hips and thighs are wider
than chest and shoulders;
appearance is bottom-heavy

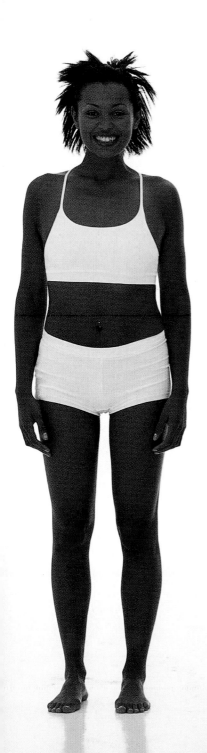
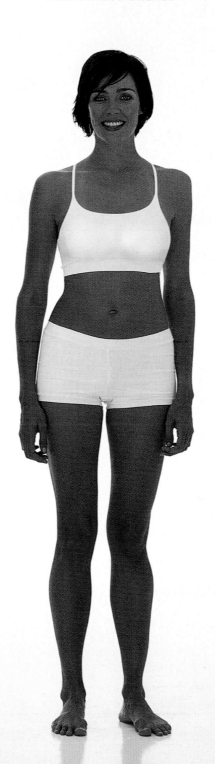
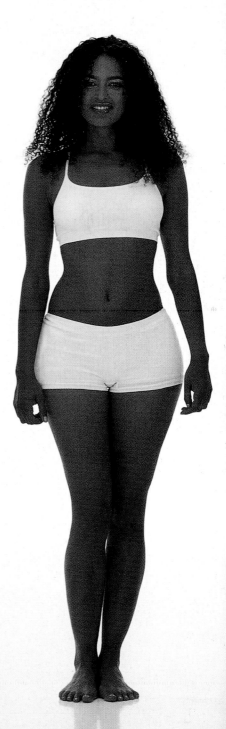

tube body profile

The tube is possibly the most envied and desired of all the body shapes. It is simply human nature to want what we don't have. Voluptuous women yearn for a straight-up-and-down figure; those who are as straight as a ruler hanker after a curvaceous, shapely one.

The tube-shaped woman has a small waist, narrow hips, and a small rear end. Although these may be exactly the features that apples, pears, and hourglasses desire, many women with this shape feel they lack sufficient form to show their body to its best advantage.

This is not to say that you should see your tubular shape as something to be ashamed of—in fact, quite the reverse. While it's unlikely that you'll ever be as curvaceous as the hourglass, you have a distinct advantage in being the easiest shape to work with. Keep this positive thought in mind as you follow my recommended combination of workouts.

the tube

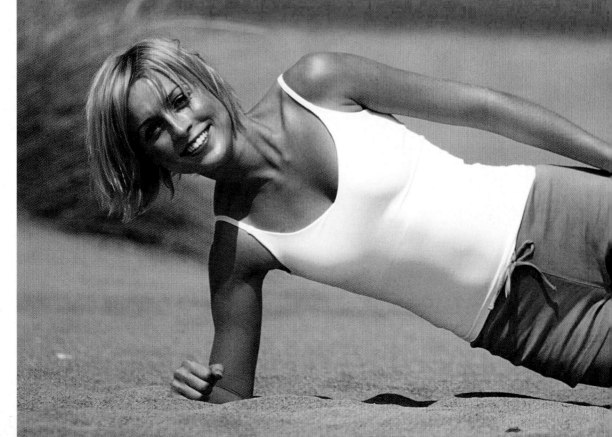

your special features

Upper body
The continuing theme for this body shape is its lack of curves. The upper body tends to be relatively square, with a small chest and back.

Arms
Like the legs, the arms may be long and thin, but without definition or apparent strength. Strong arms with good muscle tone have a curious way of making the whole body look fitter, taller, and more curvaceous.

Hips and thighs
The hip area is rarely wider than the waist or shoulders. The lean thighs often lack shape.

Waist
A particular characteristic of the tube's figure is that there tends to be little or even no definition around the waist area—the torso is literally straight up and down. This can make the overall body shape appear shorter or wider than it really is.

Lower body
Long, lean, and often with little excess body fat, the tube shape usually boasts a slender lower half, right down to the feet. By creating muscle definition in the thighs and calves, and toning the ankles, the legs will appear even longer and more elegant.

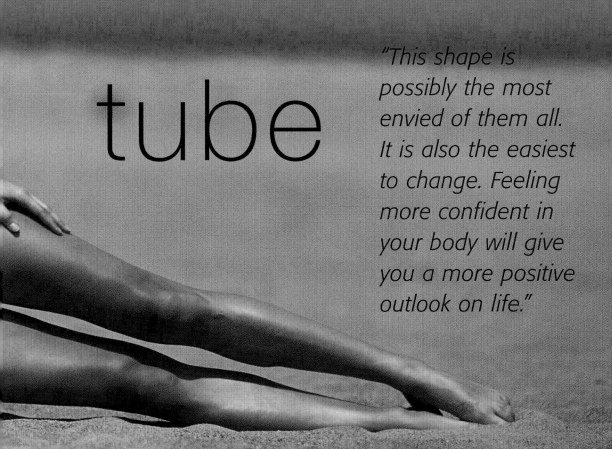

tube

"This shape is possibly the most envied of them all. It is also the easiest to change. Feeling more confident in your body will give you a more positive outlook on life."

your body shape at a glance

Upper body

- Shoulders are narrow and tend to slump forward.
- Arms are lean and often lacking in shape and tone.
- Chest tends to be relatively flat.
- Upper back needs definition to create the appearance of depth and strength.

Middle body

- Waistline and lower back do not curve in as they do in the other body shapes.
- Waist area is usually lean, but without much definition.
- There is very little difference between the waist and hip measurements.

Lower body

- Small and usually well toned, the tube's rear end is an object of envy for many women. Lower body exercises help to create a more rounded appearance.
- Legs are long and slender, with lean thighs and little definition in the calves.

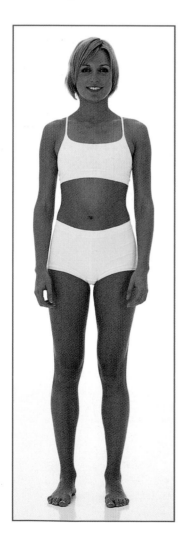

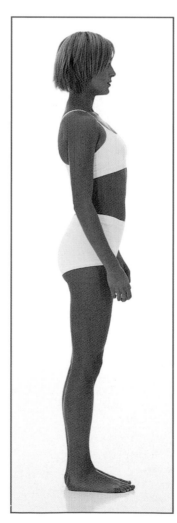

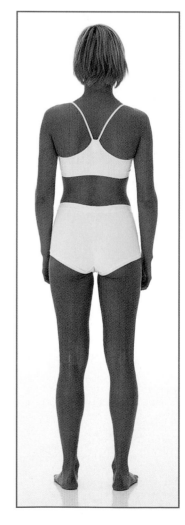

the tube

Workout goals

Develop strong, well-defined shoulders Enhancing the upper body helps create the illusion of curves—wider shoulders leading to a small waist.

Tone arms and build up body strength Tube shapes are lucky to have slender arms, but they lack shape and definition. To build up strength and muscle tone in the upper body area, we'll be doing workouts with dumbbells and high repetitions.

Accentuate your waistline As we're creating a V-shape by working the shoulder and chest area, we'll help accentuate this by ensuring the stomach is strong and flat.

Create a bottom A lack of lower body curves can make you appear shapeless. We'll aim for a sexy, womanly rear to make your legs look even longer and leaner.

The single arm shoulder press helps to build strength in the upper body. It is extra effective when done with dumbbells. See page 51 for full instructions.

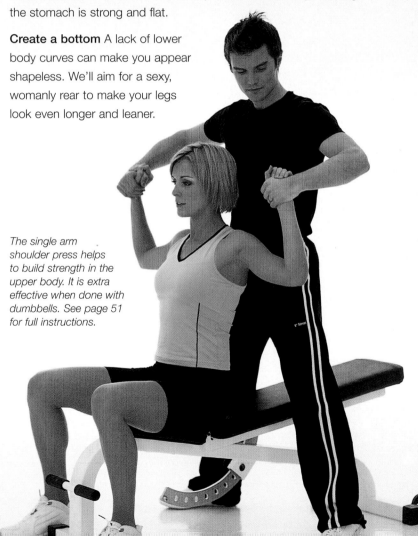

Let's get started

Read the introduction to the workouts for your shape, then do the step-by-step exercises. As your fitness level improves, you can increase the reps or duration of the workout, or add dumbbells where appropriate.

- **gym: workout 1** *(page 36):* to elongate, strengthen, and tone the upper body.
- **gym: workout 2** *(page 58):* to create definition in the upper body.
- **gym: workout 3** *(page 76):* high-repetition workout to burn fat and calories.
- **home: workout 6** *(page 136):* feel the burn and get your heart pumping.

For optimum results, try this workout program:

Day 1   gym: workout 1
Day 2   rest
Day 3   gym: workout 2
Day 4   rest
Day 5   gym: workout 3
Day 6   home: workout 6
Day 7   rest

eat well, look great

Healthy eating for your shape

Good news for tube shapes: you have more latitude than any other body shape when it comes to eating what you want. Just remember not to go overboard. To support your workout program, it's important to include carbohydrates in your daily diet. While you should still avoid "white" carbohydrates—for example, white bread, pasta and rice—their whole-wheat and unprocessed counterparts are acceptable. Try to include a small amount of protein in each meal. However, a predominantly protein-based diet can encourage your body to consume its energy resources—leaving it thin but nevertheless unhealthy.

Energy level maintenance

Aim to eat some form of complex carbohydrates before and after your workout, to help fuel your body and replace lost energy. Without this slow-release energy source, you may feel lethargic and listless because your body shape tends to metabolize food quite quickly. To maintain optimum energy, try to eat small meals regularly. This will keep your blood sugar level stable, helping you to avoid energy dips and the familiar afternoon slump, when you are more likely to reach for a sweet snack to give yourself a boost.

"Tube shapes tend to metabolize food quite quickly. This means that they can lose weight even when eating a healthy, balanced diet, and may even be underweight."

What to wear to make the most of your shape

Many women would do just about anything to get your figure, so show it off to its best advantage.

- Wear loose knits and flowing fabrics that skim and soften your shape.
- Select styles that help to define your waistline, such as drawstring pants or elastic-waisted skirts.
- Cinch in your waist with a slender belt.
- Go monochrome: one color from neck to hem is extremely elegant.
- Sport colorful scarves and jewelry to draw attention to your slender neckline.

Avoid these

- Boxy jackets, which reinforce your straight-up-and-down shape.
- Very tailored styles, unless you want to look severe.
- Wide-leg, full, or voluminous trousers—they emphasize the lack of curves.

the tube

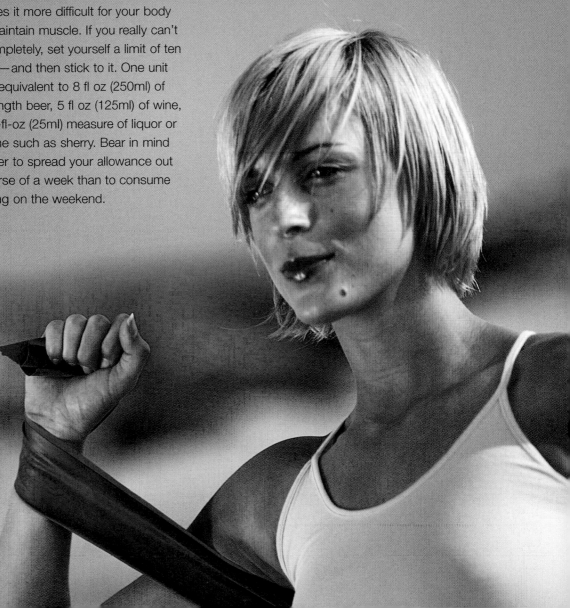

Counting the calories

Tube shapes may have difficulty keeping their weight stable and are frequently underweight. To help maintain your body weight or even to gain weight, you will need to eat around 2,200–2,400 calories a day. It is particularly important to provide your body with enough fuel while following an exercise program.

A word about alcohol

Try to avoid alcohol while you are training. Alcohol makes it more difficult for your body to build or maintain muscle. If you really can't cut it out completely, set yourself a limit of ten units a week—and then stick to it. One unit of alcohol is equivalent to 8 fl oz (250ml) of average-strength beer, 5 fl oz (125ml) of wine, or a single 1-fl-oz (25ml) measure of liquor or a fortified wine such as sherry. Bear in mind that it is better to spread your allowance out over the course of a week than to consume it in one sitting on the weekend.

10 foods to enjoy

Whole-wheat pasta	Sweet potatoes
Whole-wheat bread	Squash
Eggplant	Peas
Mangoes	Sweet corn
Potatoes	Carrots

apple body profile

Of all the body shapes, the apple perhaps carries the most negative connotations. The very word conjures up images of a shapeless, dumpy body, with no tone or strength. On the contrary, the apple is one of the most common female body shapes, and has many positive attributes.

The apple definition is given to this shape because the upper body dimensions are somewhat larger and rounder than the lower body. The shoulders, back, and chest are proportionately larger than the hips and thighs, thereby creating the rounded, applelike effect. Instead of trying to reduce the size of your upper body, our aim will be to strengthen and tone your chest, arms, and upper back. To balance the upper and lower body, we will also focus on your midsection, hips, thighs, calves, and ankles. Within a few weeks, your body will start to look better balanced and more streamlined.

the apple

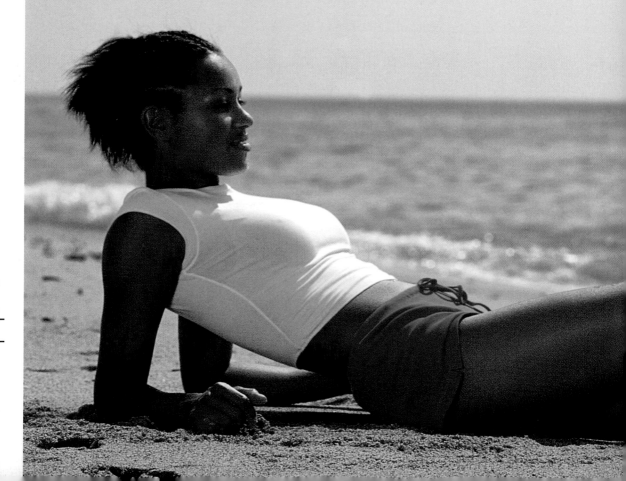

your special features

Arms
The apple has well-shaped arms, but the upper arms may be flabby. The wrists and forearms are comparatively delicate.

Chest
The chest area is large, giving the typically top-heavy look. Although this is the first place the apple tends to put on weight, it is also the easiest place from which to lose it.

Upper and lower back
The broad, strong back of the apple has a tendency to retain weight and look heavy.

Waist and stomach
The waist is more or less defined depending on the underlying muscle tone. As with the back, the waist and stomach tend to store body fat, and this can make the apple body look bulkier than it actually is, even if not overweight.

Hips, rear, and legs
The lower body of the apple is usually a real asset—one that the pear would love to have. The hips are narrow in proportion to the width of the shoulders, the backside is small and flat, and the legs are lean but shapely. These help to give the apple a graceful appearance.

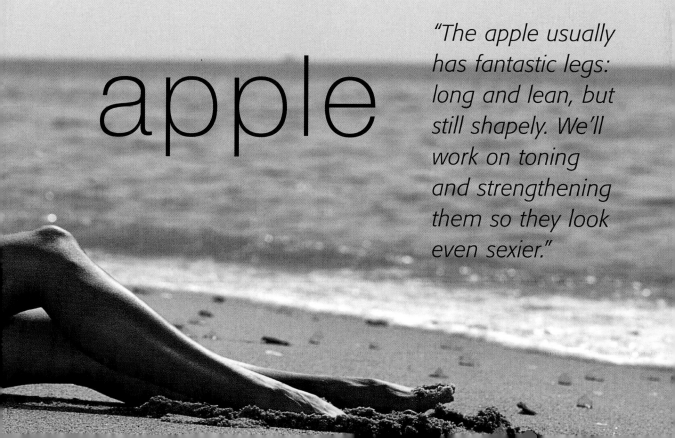

apple

"The apple usually has fantastic legs: long and lean, but still shapely. We'll work on toning and strengthening them so they look even sexier."

your body shape at a glance

Upper body

- Shoulders are proportionately wider than the hips.
- Upper arms often lack tone.
- Chest area is generous and is somewhat out of proportion to the lower body.
- Upper back is broad and strong but may be fleshy.

Middle body

- Waistline, when toned, is lean and has some definition.
- Waist and abdomen tend to accumulate excess body fat. The whole shape looks larger than it really is if the stomach area is slack and paunchy.
- Waist is similar in width to hips.

Lower body

- Hips and thighs are usually small in proportion to the upper body.
- Thighs are lean and rarely carry excess body fat.
- Skinny or bony ankles can make legs look almost too thin.
- Rear end is small and flat, or virtually nonexistent.

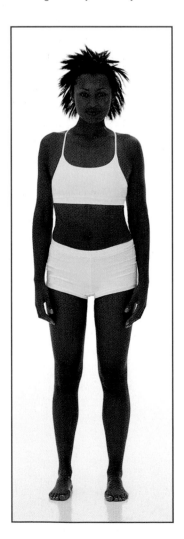
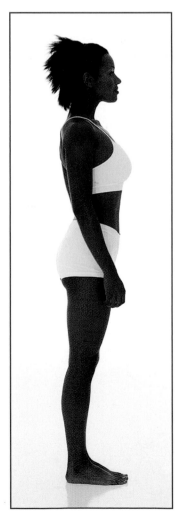
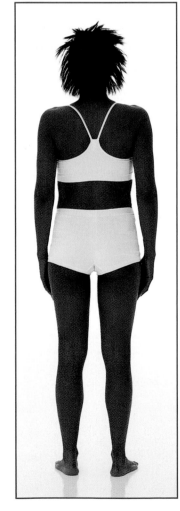

the apple

Workout goals

Reduce body fat Women with a typical apple shape store excess weight around their waist and stomach. We'll be doing high-intensity, fat-burning exercises to create a flat and fabulous tummy.

Use your muscles Fat-burning programs use aerobic exercises. We will also engage the larger muscles of the upper body to help burn fat from the arms, chest, and midriff, and define the upper back.

Tone and strengthen the upper body The apple body boasts a strong, wide chest and upper back area. We'll concentrate on defining and balancing your upper body with your lower half.

Increase the workout intensity Aerobic exercises raise your heart rate and your metabolic rate so that your body burns fat faster. This will help in our aim to give your body better visual proportions.

Emphasize your good points The apple shape has fabulous legs. We'll make them better than ever with exercises that work on your thighs, calves, and ankles.

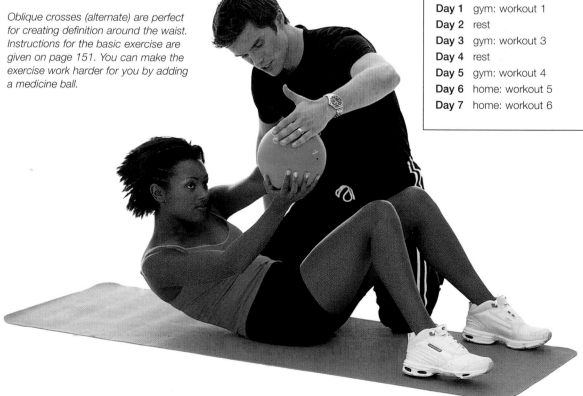

Oblique crosses (alternate) are perfect for creating definition around the waist. Instructions for the basic exercise are given on page 151. You can make the exercise work harder for you by adding a medicine ball.

Let's get started

Read the introduction to the workouts for your shape, then do the step-by-step exercises. As your fitness level improves, you can increase the reps or duration of the workout, or add dumbbells where appropriate.

- **gym: workout 1** *(page 36)*: to elongate, strengthen, and tone the upper body.
- **gym: workout 3** *(page 76)*: high-repetition workout to burn fat and calories.
- **gym: workout 4** *(page 98)*: for upper body definition.
- **home: workout 5** *(page 116)*: to burn calories and reduce body fat.
- **home workout 6** *(page 136)*: feel the burn and get your heart pumping.

For optimum results, try this workout program:

Day 1   gym: workout 1
Day 2   rest
Day 3   gym: workout 3
Day 4   rest
Day 5   gym: workout 4
Day 6   home: workout 5
Day 7   home: workout 6

eat well, look great

Healthy eating for your shape

Whatever your shape, I advise eating foods mainly from the low to medium end of the glycemic index (for more about this, turn to pages 26 and 32). This is particularly sound advice for the apple shape, with its tendency to store excess body fat on the waistline and stomach. It will also help to reduce digestive stress—a common problem for apples. Before beginning this new way of eating, follow my bloat-busting guidelines for two weeks.

Bloat-busting guidelines

Avoid wheat-based products. Many people have an intolerance to wheat, and it is a major cause of bloating. Avoid cow's milk and other dairy products. These also irritate a sensitive digestive system. Experiment instead with milk from nondairy sources such as soy or rice. (After two weeks, you can slowly reintroduce wheat and dairy products into your diet, one meal at a time, if you wish.) Never go without breakfast. Try oatmeal made with water, or rye-bread toast with a little jam but no butter. Have some non-citrus fruit such as dates, plums, or kiwi fruit, or make a fresh fruit smoothie.

"To help prevent bloating, I recommend that you eliminate wheat and dairy products from your diet for two weeks. You'll be amazed at how different you look and feel."

What to wear to make the most of your shape

Elongate a top-heavy, rounded figure with these clever dressing tricks.

- Wear all one color to create an illusion of height.
- Choose tailored pants with straight or tapered legs.
- Play up the neatness of your hips with slim or streamlined skirts.
- Wear shorter skirts with nude hosiery to draw attention down to your legs.
- Try unstructured jackets, but make sure they fit well (no slouchy shoulderline).
- Go for fine fabrics such as cotton, cashmere, and light wool.

Avoid these

- Very fitted jackets—they'll accentuate your larger top half.
- Thick or bulky sweaters.
- Anything double-breasted.

the apple

Lunch suggestions

Have a salad made with your choice of: chickpeas, cooked or canned butter beans, lentils, brown rice, wild rice, millet, grated raw carrot, grated zucchini, apple, red or orange peppers, avocado, beets. Dress with a little virgin olive oil and a squeeze of orange or lemon juice, and add some fresh herbs if you like. If it's a cold day or you need cheering up, try a nondairy soup made with lots of vegetables.

Evening meal suggestions

Steamed or poached fish or grilled chicken breast are good choices when you're giving your stomach a rest. Serve with lightly cooked vegetables. Try to experiment with different kinds, including the more unusual ones, such as sweet potatoes, to liven up your mealtime. This will help you avoid "boredom eating," which can occur when you are following a restricted eating plan.

Snack suggestions

I'm a firm believer in snacks. In their own way, they are as important as main meals because they keep your energy level stable and stop you from reaching for a sugary treat. Just be selective. Try raw carrot sticks, grapes, orchard fruits such as apples or pears, or a small handful of pumpkin or sunflower seeds.

10 foods to enjoy

Red peppers	Carrots
Parsnips	Pears
Celery	Fresh dates
Mushrooms	Papaya
Squash	Kiwi fruit

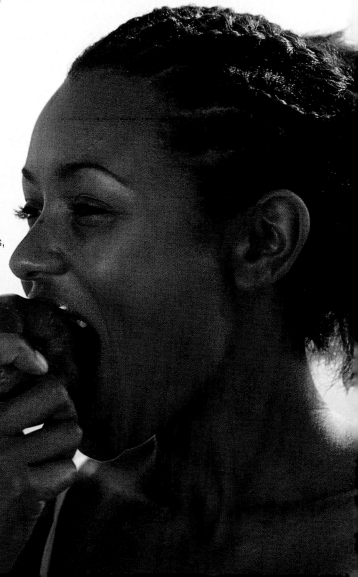

hourglass body profile

The timeless allure of the classic female figure is seen in the hourglass shape, and it's no better represented than by the Hollywood screen goddesses and icons of the 1950s. Jayne Mansfield, Marilyn Monroe and other "blonde bombshells"— they had all the right curves in all the right places, and are surely the epitome of what can be achieved with an hourglass body.

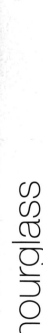

So it's a pity that this curvaceous, womanly shape is one that is often not wholly liked by those who possess it. Perhaps the negative associations stem from the fact that it can be a difficult shape to dress, particularly if the body is carrying excess weight. Then, the curves may seem almost out of control. The real key to creating a fabulous hourglass shape is to ensure that the natural slimness of the waistline is maximized, and that the upper and lower body curves are toned, sculpted, and well-proportioned.

your special features

Shoulders and chest
The shoulders are often reasonably wide and need little work. However, the rear part of the shoulder and the supporting muscles around the shoulder blades should be used to encourage a "pulling back" and "lifting" of the chest to increase the curvaceous look.

Upper and lower back
Good posture is vital to ensure that the curves appear evenly balanced, and to open up the waistline to its full potential. We will spend a considerable amount of time on this area. The lower back plays a crucial role in lifting the pelvis and creating a shapely rear. It is this definition that will balance the curves and prevent the backside from "slumping" over the backs of the legs.

Arms
Hourglass arms usually require some toning and definition, but it is important to achieve this without increasing the bulk.

Waist
This is the best feature, so we'll make sure it stays that way. We are going to sculpt and tone the waistline for a sexy, curvaceous, and very feminine shape.

Hips, rear, and legs
Here is where the hourglass curves may tend to go out of control. As with the shoulders, the hips are reasonably wide, and the backside is proportionately generous. Thighs are shapely but usually in need of some work to improve the underlying muscle tone.

the hourglass

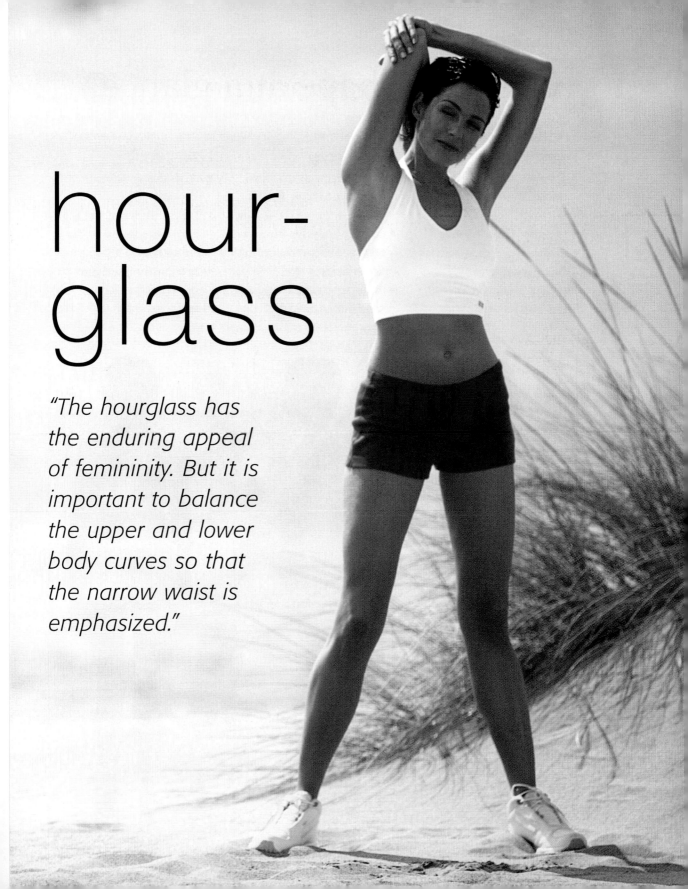

hour-glass

"The hourglass has the enduring appeal of femininity. But it is important to balance the upper and lower body curves so that the narrow waist is emphasized."

eat well, look great

Healthy eating for your shape

The bulk of your diet should consist of foods from the low to medium end of the glycemic index. (The glycemic index, or GI, is a system that rates the carbohydrate content of foods on a scale of high to low.) High GI foods release their energy quickly, which also raises your blood sugar level. This gives the energy high that is followed by the corresponding low. It's only natural then to reach for a sweet snack in order to achieve a similar "high," and so the vicious circle is repeated. I hope this will help you to understand that it really does make sense to eat mostly low to medium GI foods (see below). Then you can allow yourself the occasional treat of a (preferably low-fat) high GI food such as bananas or cheese.

Low to medium GI foods

Eating a low GI diet will also help to reduce any tendency to accumulate fat on the hips and thighs. Most fruits (except bananas), vegetables, legumes, beans, grains, and seeds are fine. For non-vegetable protein, choose fish or the white meat of chicken; oily fish such as fresh tuna is a good addition to your diet. Limit your intake of dairy products. Especially avoid refined sugar, processed foods, and white bread, potatoes, pasta, and rice.

"Don't let your natural hourglass curves get out of hand. Base your diet on seasonal vegetables, fruits, and low-fat protein: it's a delicious and healthy way to tame them."

the hourglass

What to wear to make the most of your shape

The secret is in the proportions. A toned and sculpted hourglass looks fantastic in most outfits.

- Choose clothes that emphasize the narrowness of your waist. Smartly tailored suits are perfect for formal wear, or try structured jackets and slim skirts.
- Acquire a collection of belts. Thin ones are best if you are short.
- Invest in the best quality underwear you can afford.

Avoid these

- Unstructured, loose, or baggy garments. They will hide your curves and make your body look stocky and inelegant.

Counting the calories

A well-proportioned hourglass figure should stay that way with exercise and a healthy, balanced diet of mostly fruit, vegetables, legumes, and grains. If you find counting calories useful, aim for 2,500 calories a day. Whether or not you're counting them, limit your fat intake to no more than 30g a day.

A word about alcohol

While training, avoid alcohol, or limit yourself to ten units spread out over the week. One unit of alcohol is equivalent to 8 fl oz (250ml) of average-strength beer, 5 fl oz (125ml) of wine, or a single 1-fl-oz (25ml) measure of liquor or a fortified wine such as sherry.

10 foods to enjoy

Broccoli	Melons
Cabbage	Pineapple
Asparagus	Strawberries
Mushrooms	Wild rice
Spinach	Butter beans
Chicory	Sesame seeds

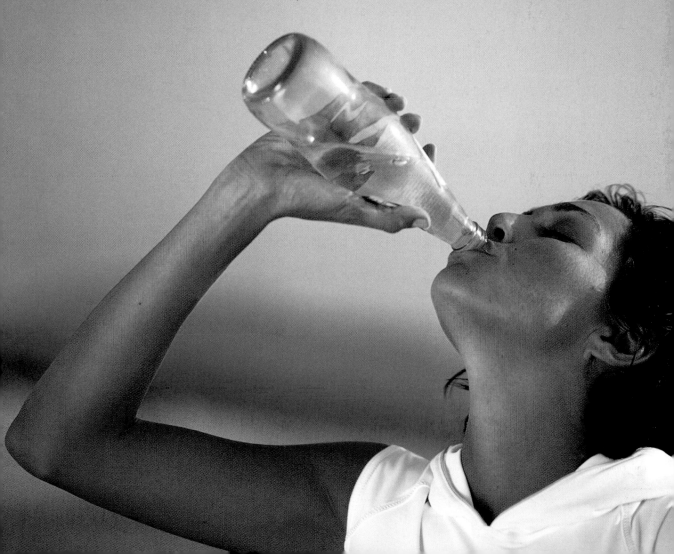

pear body profile

The pear is possibly the body shape that is most disliked by those who possess it. Often referred to as the classic English shape, it is actually very common in other cultures, and is a shape seen among women of oriental and African descent as well as western European.

Within the history of the female form, the pear shape has been not so much derided as admired because of its visual association with fertility and childbirth. The pear's most obvious feature are the hips. Typically wider than those of the tube, apple, and hourglass, it is the hips that give the pear-shaped woman the appearance of being better suited to child-bearing than the other body shapes. Sadly, although a wide pelvis may make childbirth easier, there is no evidence to suggest that the pear actually is more fertile than the other shapes.

your special features

Arms
The pear tends to have long, elegant arms, although they can be lacking in shape and definition. Fortunately, arms respond well to exercise, and are one of the easiest areas to strengthen and tone.

Shoulders and upper back
These are definitely one of the pear's best features. The shoulders are narrow and the slim upper back carries little body fat, giving this area a very svelte appearance. However, the relative narrowness may accentuate the generous hips and rear, and make them seem larger than they really are.

Hips and thighs
This is the part of the body that causes the pear shape most concern. Typically, excess body fat is held from just above the hips (or sometimes from below the ribs in the upper back) down to the tops of the thighs. Although it is important not to overwork this area, there is hope, since it responds well to exercise.

Rear end
In profile, the pear's bottom seems almost to merge into the upper thighs. As with the hips and thighs, the appropriate exercises will help to lift the buttocks so that the whole body has a more sculpted and shapely appearance.

the pear

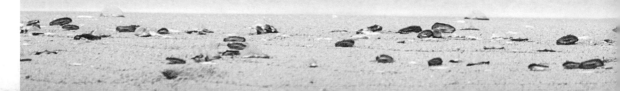

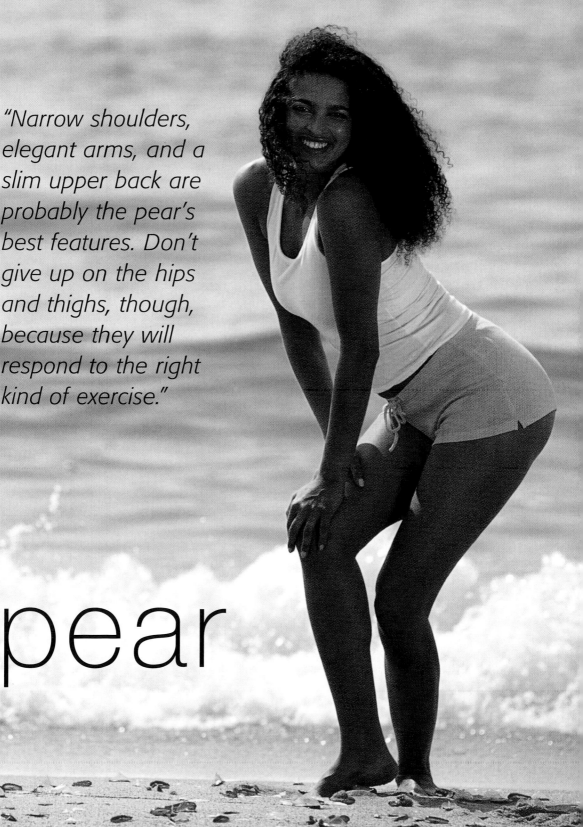

"Narrow shoulders, elegant arms, and a slim upper back are probably the pear's best features. Don't give up on the hips and thighs, though, because they will respond to the right kind of exercise."

pear

your body shape at a glance

Upper body

- Shoulders are narrow but may look rounded because the posture tends to slump forward.
- Chest is often rather slim, with relatively small breasts.
- In terms of measurement, the chest is in proportion to the narrow shoulders.

Middle body

- Waistline is well defined, although this area and the lower back can carry excess fat.
- Stomach may look flabby with poor underlying muscle tone. This can make the whole body look overweight even if it is not carrying excess fat.

Lower body

- Hips and rear are wider than the shoulders, which creates the classic pear shape. The rear end is long rather than pert, seeming to disappear into the thighs.
- Thighs are rounded to chunky, although the lower legs tend to be shapely with trim ankles.

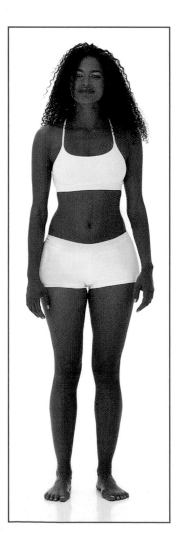
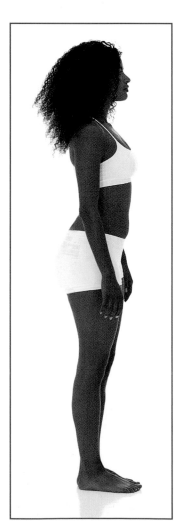
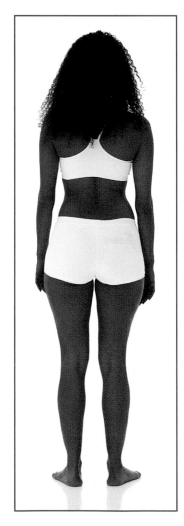

the pear

Workout goals

Develop strong, well-defined shoulders By strengthening and visually widening the upper body, we will create a better balance between the shoulders and hips.

Accentuate the form of the upper back This is one of your best features. Exercises that concentrate on improving the underlying muscle structure will give the added benefit of improved posture. Standing strong and upright creates a taller, slimmer silhouette.

Reduce fat on the hips, rear, and thighs The focus will be on exercises that help to reduce any excess body fat stored here. Too often, women with pear-shaped figures spend hours doing lower body work, which just builds mass in the hips and thighs. Instead, we'll slim down the area to create a new shapeliness in the rear end and define the curve between buttocks and thighs.

Fitness ball hamstring curls are one of the most efficient exercises for strengthening and toning the backs of the thighs. Instructions are given on page 49.

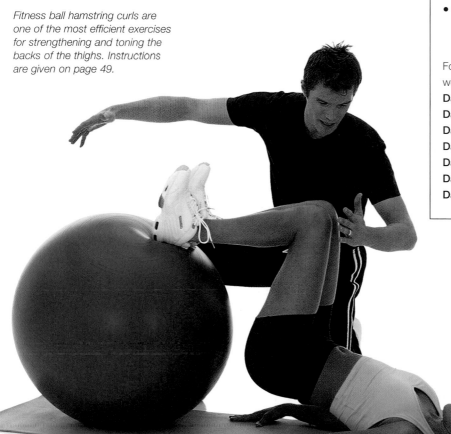

Let's get started

Read the introduction to the workouts for your shape, then do the step-by-step exercises. As your fitness level improves, you can increase the reps or duration of the workout, or add dumbbells as appropriate.

- **gym: workout 1** *(page 36):* to elongate, sculpt, and tone the whole body.
- **gym: workout 2** *(page 58):* to create definition in the upper body.
- **gym: workout 3** *(page 76):* high-repetition workout to burn fat and calories.
- **gym: workout 4** *(page 98):* for upper body definition.
- **home: workout 6** *(page 136):* feel the burn and get your heart pumping.

For optimum results, try this workout program

Day 1 gym: workout 1
Day 2 rest
Day 3 gym: workout 2
Day 4 rest
Day 5 gym: workout 3
Day 6 gym: workout 4
Day 7 home: workout 6

eat well, look great

Healthy eating for your shape

You may already know that I recommend eating mainly from the low to medium end of the glycemic index or GI—the system that rates the carbohydrate component of foods from high to low. Read on, and you'll understand the wisdom in this. Foods (such as mashed potato) that are rated high on the GI scale contain carbohydrates that are quickly broken down in the body to enter the bloodstream as glucose (the speed at which this occurs is what causes the energy rush that is typically followed by an energy dip). The faster glucose enters the bloodstream, the more insulin your body makes. High levels of insulin stop your body from using stored body fat for energy. So if your diet contains a large proportion of high GI foods, you'll have a tendency to put on weight or find it hard to maintain your ideal weight.

Raw foods to lose fat, boost energy

Eating raw foods reduces toxins in the body, which in turn reduces the amount of fat stored. As your body begins to function more efficiently, you'll feel an increase in energy, too. This doesn't mean you have to munch your way through platefuls of raw carrots. Just make sure that your main meal always includes a selection of raw or lightly cooked vegetables.

"Cutting down on food encourages the body to store fat. Eat plenty of fresh fruit, vegetables, and grains plus some lean protein to reach and maintain your ideal weight."

What to wear to make the most of your shape

The trick is to display your best features and camouflage the areas you're still working on.

- Choose tailored, long-line jackets that fall below your rear end. Wide lapels or interesting detail at the neck will draw the eye naturally upward.
- Use belts to accentuate a well-defined waist, but don't cinch them in too tightly or your lower half will look disproportionately large.
- Experiment with eye-catching earrings and necklaces.
- Wear solid colors rather than patterns on your lower body.

Avoid these

- Very short skirts—they will make your legs look shorter and your hips wider.
- Any outfit that is too small, tight, or revealing.

the pear

Counting the calories

If you need to lose weight, aim for no more than 1,800 calories a day. Once you have reached your target weight, you'll need about 2,200 calories a day to maintain this level of muscle tone and body fat. Remember, though, that muscle weighs more than fat, and that the fit of your clothes may tell you more than the scales.

Carbohydrates bad and good

Limit your intake of carbohydrates from the high end of the GI scale, including white bread, pasta and rice, potatoes, parsnips, bananas, red meat, honey and other sugars, and processed foods. Enjoy those from the low to medium end of the scale. Most vegetables (including sweet potatoes) are fine, as are beans, lentils, grains, and seeds.

A word about alcohol

There is no nutritional value in alcohol, and for the pear-shaped woman its calories soon settle around the hips, thighs, and stomach. Either cut it out or stick to ten units spread out over a week (but aim to have weeks when you are seriously under that amount). One unit of alcohol is equivalent to 8 fl oz (250ml) of average-strength beer, 5 fl oz (125ml) of wine, or a single 1-fl-oz (25ml) measure of liquor or a fortified wine such as sherry.

10 foods to enjoy

Broccoli	Carrots
Cabbage	Cauliflower
Mushrooms	Butter beans
Onions	Sesame seeds
Peppers	Wild rice

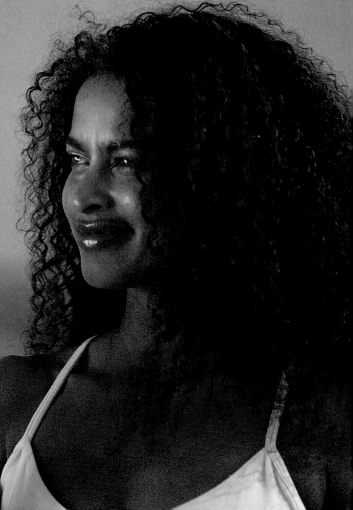

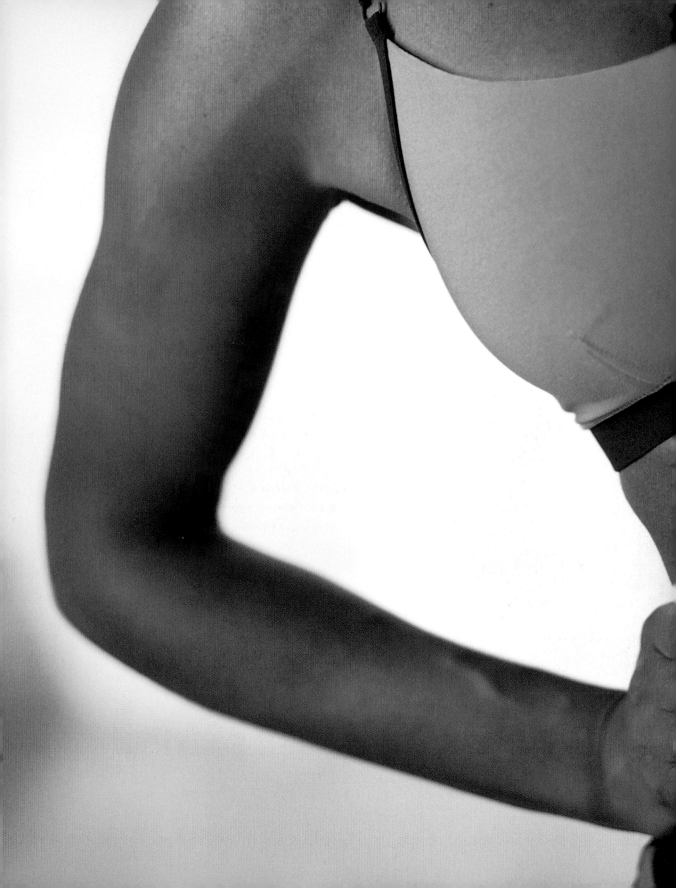

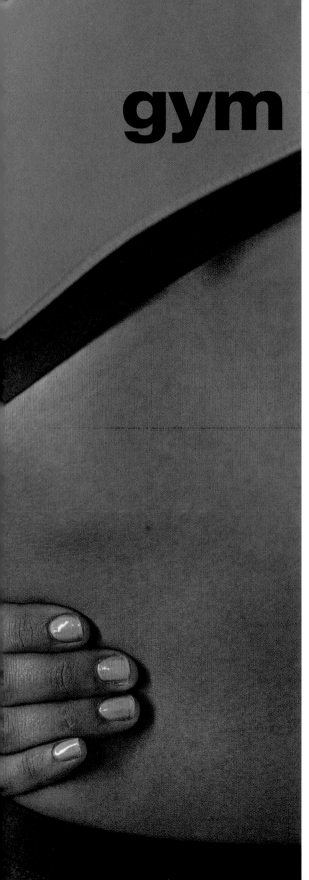

gym workouts

Now that you know what body shape you are, it's time to get moving. Making a commitment to begin a fitness program is just the first step in achieving your goals, but if you follow my motivational tips, this time your fitness program will really work.

Be in the right frame of mind Don't try to begin a fitness program if you're frantically busy. Choose a period in your schedule when you have time to dedicate to yourself and your body.

Set realistic time periods Don't be disheartened if your body shape isn't changing as quickly as you'd like. Set long-term goals and reward yourself along the way for the small successes you achieve.

Use clear measuring guides Never, ever weigh yourself when it comes to assessing your progress. Use the fit of your clothes, your eyes, and the way you feel about your body as a realistic measure of your achievement. If you really must, use a measuring tape to record the changes occurring in your body.

Make yourself a priority Sticking to your workout schedule is just as important as keeping a business or social appointment. You are just as important as anybody else, so write down "when," "where," and "what" you will be doing on a specific day, and do it.

Be positive You're going to have some days when you don't feel like exercising. Remind yourself of your achievements—and how much better you'll feel once you've honored the commitment to yourself.

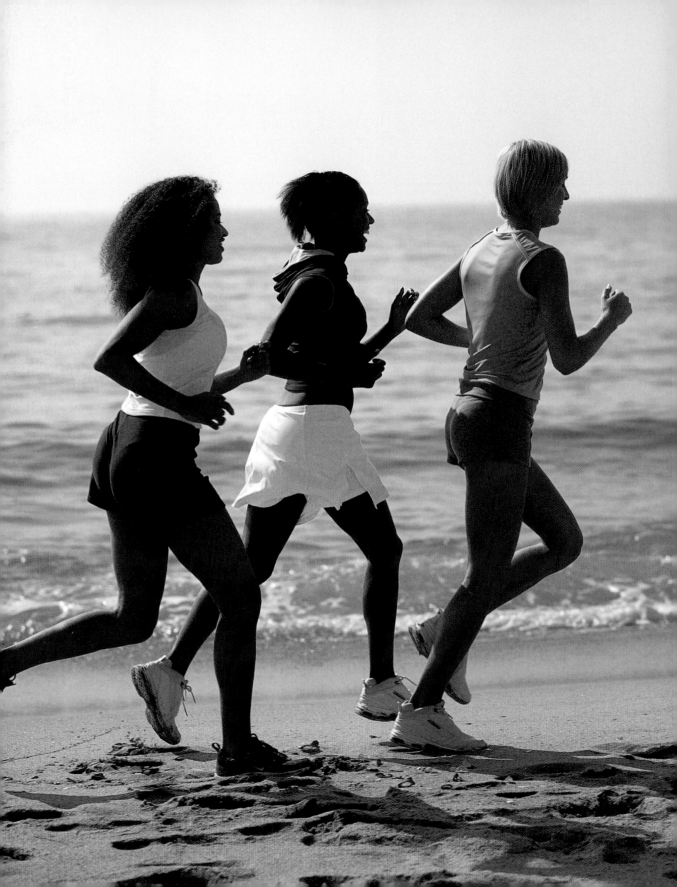

sculpt and tone 1

This program is called a peripheral heart action (PHA) workout. By alternating between the upper and lower body, we'll achieve fantastic fat-burning results.

This program is an ideal way for tube, apple, and pear shapes to achieve their exercise goals. As the workout switches between the upper and lower body, it burns fat quickly and effectively. This is because the heart and lungs have to work harder to provide blood to all areas of the body, so you'll be burning an extremely large number of calories due to the effort required. As well as burning fat, you will also benefit from the overall toning and conditioning of every muscle group. This will streamline your body, and reduce overall body "mass" in all areas. It also helps reduce fat around the problem areas such as hips, backside, and thighs for pears, enhances shape and curves for tube shapes, and reduces the upper body size in apples.

gym: workout 1

exercise	perform	exercise	perform
cross trainer	6 min	rower	⅓ mile (500m)
rower	⅓ mile (500m)	single arm shoulder press	20 reps per side
straight arm pulldowns	15 reps	step-ups	25 reps per side
walking lunge	20 lunges	lateral raise (slow)	15 reps
seated leg curl	15 reps	wide leg squat	20 reps
hill walk	3 min	single arm lateral raise	15 reps per side
close grip pulldowns	15 reps	cross trainer	3 min
alternating power lunge	30 reps	*repeat the workout starting from the*	
single arm bent over row	20 reps per side	*straight arm pulldowns*	
fitness ball hamstring curl	25 reps	*cool-down stretches as prescribed*	

cross trainer

A cross trainer is a great way to warm up your body and get your heart pumping strongly. This encourages your body to burn fat, and improves your overall fitness.

Do 6 minutes

1 Stand firmly on the pedals and program in the required information, including your height and weight. Set the machine for 6 minutes, and the maximum heart rate (MHR) to 80%.

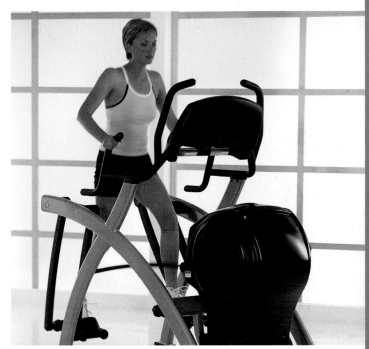

2 Gripping the handles, begin by moving your feet forward and backward. Remember to keep the pressure on your legs even. Stand up straight and keep your stomach flat and rear end under.

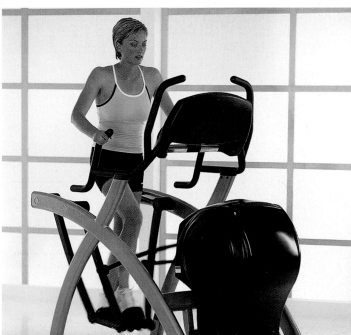

gym: warm-up 1

rower

Using a rowing machine provides high-intensity work for the upper and lower body, by raising your heart rate and burning large numbers of calories.

Do ⅓ mile (500m) at a steady pace

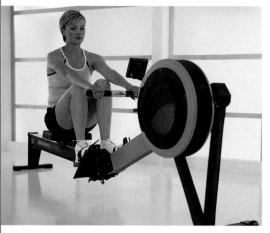

1 Your legs should be bent, with the knees tucked in close to the chest. Keep your arms straight, extended directly in front of you at shoulder level. Grip the handles firmly, with your hands positioned directly above your toes. Your torso should tilt forward slightly while your back is held firm.

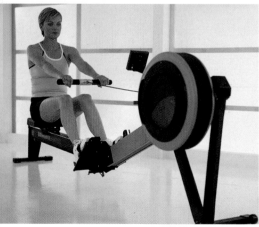

2 Start the first stroke by straightening your legs, using your leg muscles to power the movement with your arms extended in front of you. Keep your torso in the catch position as you start to pull back. Keep your arms straight until they reach the knees, then lean back slightly, pulling the handle toward your chest.

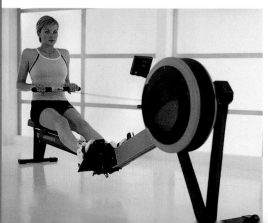

3 Pull your shoulders back so your elbows bend just behind your body. Your legs should be straight and your body tilted back slightly. As you return to the start position, stretch your arms forward and straighten them as you tilt the body forward, pivoting from the hips. As you slide forward, bend your legs and tuck your knees up close to your chest.

gym: workout 1

straight arm pulldowns

This works the muscles across the back and also the triceps, to create firm, toned upper arms. Use the cable machine with a bar attachment.

Do 15 reps

1 Stand at arm's length away from the cable machine. Facing the machine, stand with your feet hip-width apart. Take hold of the bar at shoulder-width with both hands.

2 Keeping your arms straight, pull the bar down until it reaches your thighs. Hold this position for 1 second, then return the bar to the start position.

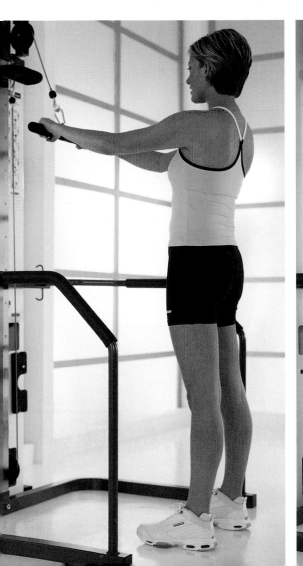

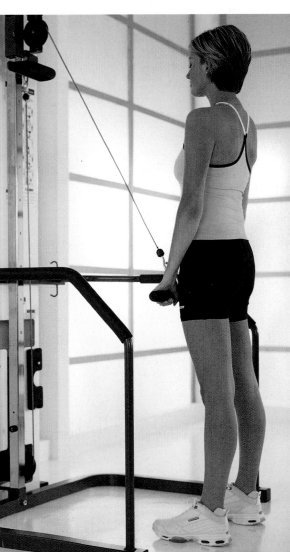

gym: workout 1

walking lunge

Unlike repetitive exercises that focus on specific muscle groups, the continuous forward movement of the walking lunge ensures greater testing of all the leg muscles. Use 11lb (5kg) dumbbells, increasing the weight with practice.

Do 20 lunges

1 Stand with feet hip-width apart and knees slightly bent. Grip the dumbbells to your sides. Using dumbbells will help you keep your balance as well as increasing the intensity of the workout.

2 Step forward about one stride-length from the back foot. In the same movement, lower your back knee toward the floor and hold for 1 second.

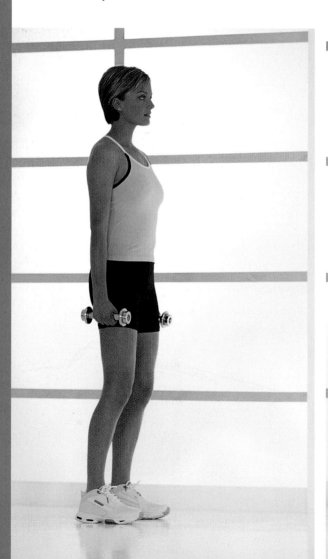
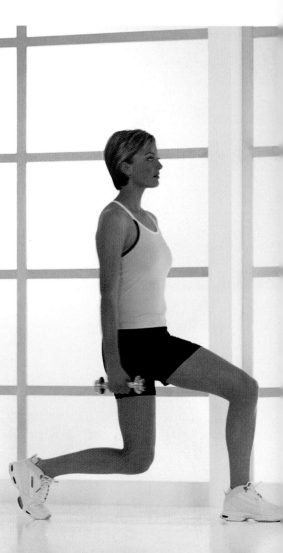

gym: workout 1

"Pears, apples, and tubes benefit from lower-body work because brings definition and tone to the hips, buttocks, and legs without adding any excess bulk."

3 Raising your body, step forward with the other leg and repeat the lunge. Keep your back straight and stomach pulled in.

4 Lower your body toward the floor. You should be focusing on ensuring that the back knee is bending straight down toward the floor. Make sure your front knee doesn't fall over your toes.

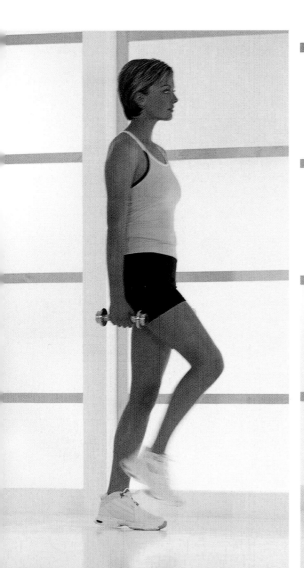

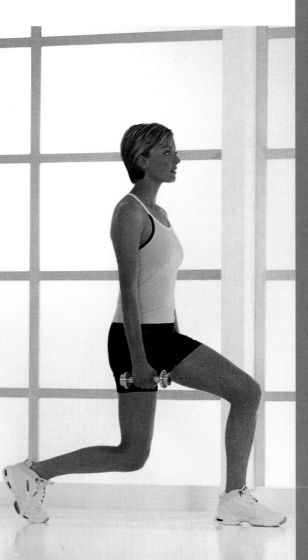

gym: workout 1

seated leg curl

Working the hamstrings—the large muscles at the backs of your thighs—creates shapely, toned legs without adding bulk to the front of the thigh. This adds shape to a tube body, and balances the upper and lower proportions of apples and pears.

Do 15 reps

1 Using the leg extension machine, sit with legs extended and your ankles on the roller pad. Keep your back at right angles to your legs. Spread the movement over 6 seconds: 3 seconds to bend the legs and 3 seconds to extend them.

2 Hold your stomach tight and bend your legs, bringing your heels toward your buttocks. Hold for a moment, then slowly return to the start position. Hold for a moment, then continue. Exhale as you lift the weights and inhale as you lower them.

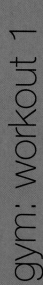

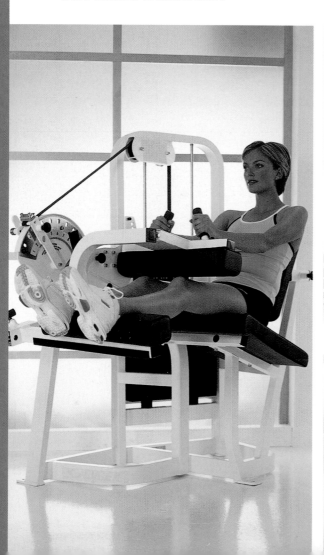

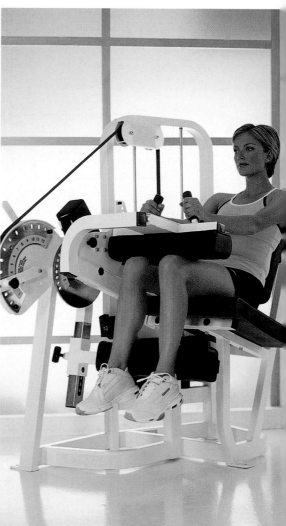

gym: workout 1

hill walk

Contrary to popular opinion, walking is as beneficial for the body as jogging. By increasing the incline on the cross trainer machine, you'll work the thighs, backs of legs, and buttocks even harder.

Set the cross trainer for 3 minutes

1 Stand firmly on the pedals and enter the required information, including your height and weight. Set the incline to at least 3. This 3-minute workout should feel like you're working your body quite hard, so adjust the resistance to ensure that you get the most out of it.

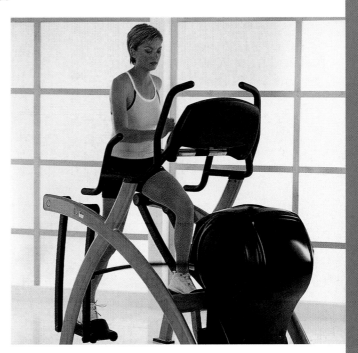

2 Keep your arms by your side and begin walking, moving the pedals forward and backward at an even pace. The movement should be controlled and even. Breathe deeply from your diaphragm.

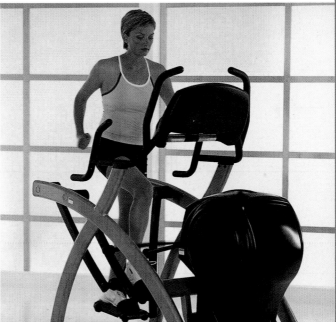

gym: workout 1

close grip pulldowns

Performing the pulldowns with a close grip works the biceps. Well-defined biceps help add definition and balance to your shape. This move is an advanced exercise and should be performed using control rather than momentum.

Do 15 reps

1 Hold the bar above your head with your hands slightly more than shoulder-width apart, using an underhand grip. Keep your back straight throughout the exercise.

2 Pull the bar down until it is at chest level. Keep your body as straight as possible. Hold for 1 second, then slowly return the bar to the start position.

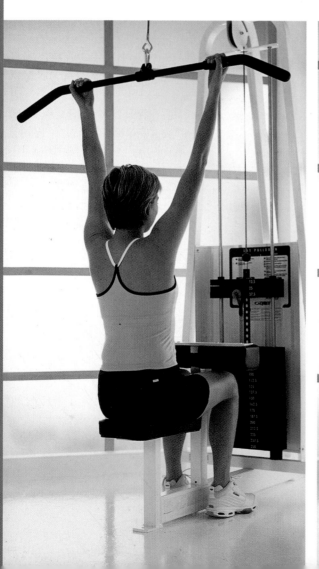

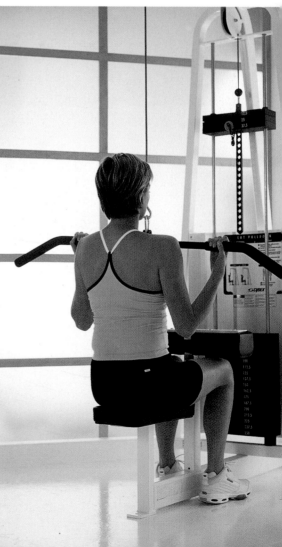

gym: workout 1

alternating power lunge

This is a more dynamic version of the lunge, but the movement should still be steady and controlled. For extra toning, pull your buttocks in tight before you start the movement.

Do 30 reps

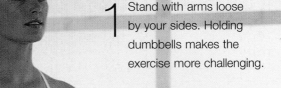

1 Stand with arms loose by your sides. Holding dumbbells makes the exercise more challenging.

2 Step forward with your left leg about 1 stride-length from the back foot, making sure that your knee does not bend farther forward than your toes. As you do so, lower your body down, then spring back to the starting position, pushing through with the heel of your front foot. Do not allow your body to waver. Now step forward with your right leg and repeat the exercise.

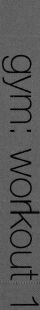

gym: workout 1

single arm bent over row

In this exercise you lift a weight toward your body, which works the biceps, back of the shoulders, and upper back. Focus on using the back muscles to pull the elbow through, rather than just relying on your biceps.

Do 20 reps on each side

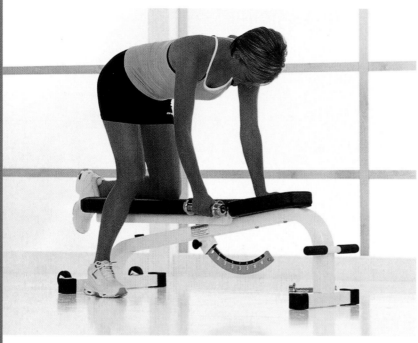

1 Rest your left hand and knee on a bench, keeping your right foot on the floor. Hold a dumbbell in your right hand so that your arm hangs down toward the floor. Keep your back straight and shoulders parallel to the floor.

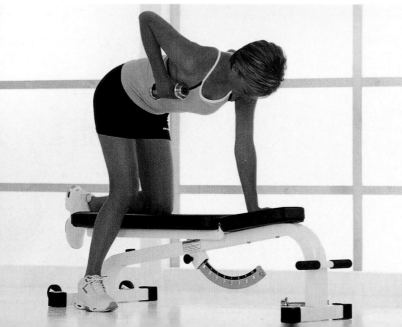

2 Pull the dumbbell up toward your chest, keeping your body stable, your back straight, and your shoulders relaxed. Keep your arm close to your body. Return to the start position, keeping the movement slow and controlled.

gym: workout 1

fitness ball hamstring curls

This is one of the best exercises for the backs of your thighs. When you get the hang of it, raise your hips off the floor in step one and then keep them raised—it makes the move even more effective.

Do 25 reps

1 Place the fitness ball against a wall, or hold it steady with your feet. Lie on your back with your arms by your sides and your palms to the floor. Rest your feet on the middle of the ball. Keep your heels hip-width apart and your toes pointing up.

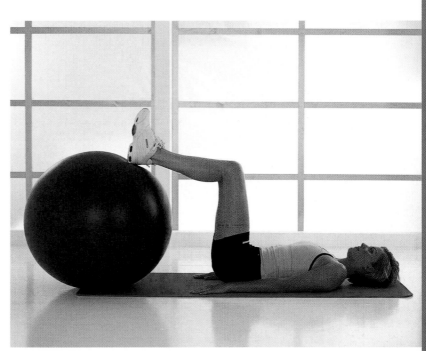

2 Gently push your heels in the top of the ball. Pull your heels slowly toward you, dragging the ball about 8in (20cm) toward you. Keep your head, shoulders, and arms still. Slowly return your legs and the ball to the start position.

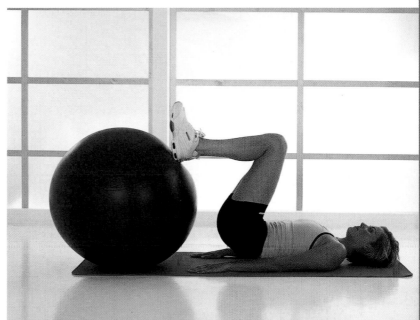

gym: workout 1

rower

Review this exercise, shown in steps on page 40. We repeat it here to increase your heart rate before beginning the next stage of the workout. Concentrate on using your legs to complete the required distance, rather than your arms.

Do ⅓ mile (500m) at a steady pace

1 Your legs should be bent. Tuck your knees in close to your chest. Keep your arms straight. Grip the handles firmly, with your hands positioned above your toes. Your torso should tilt forward slightly and your back be held firm. Straighten your leg. Use your leg muscles to power the movement.

2 Keep your arms straight until they reach your knees, then lean back slightly, pulling the handle toward your chest. Pull your shoulders back so your elbows bend just behind your body. Return to the start position. Slide forward, bend your legs, and tuck your knees close to your chest.

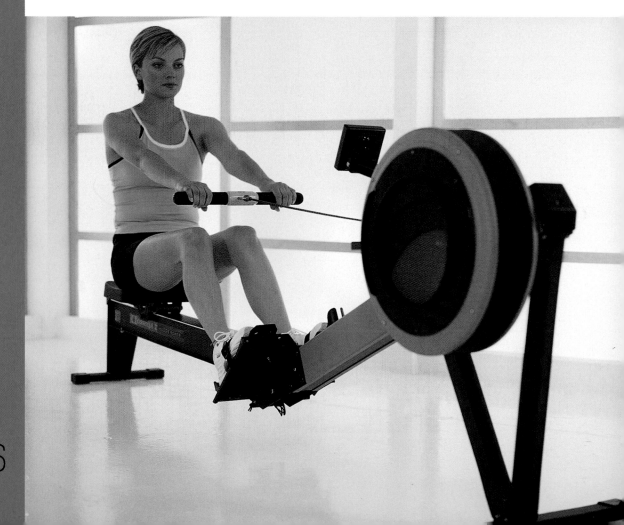

gym: workout 1

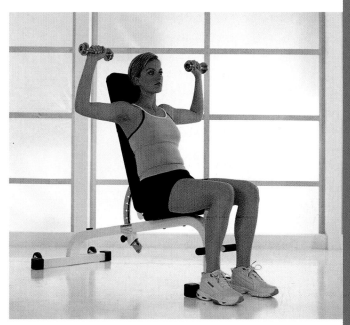

single arm shoulder press

Performing this exercise while seated focuses on the deltoids as the rest of the body is supported by the bench. If you are more advanced, you may prefer to do this exercise standing. The pressing action also works the triceps.

Do 20 reps on each side

1 Sit with your back supported by the bench, and legs bent at about 90°. Hold a weight in each hand with your arms bent at 90° and elbows out at shoulder level.

2 Keeping your left arm steady, press the weight in your right hand upward, raising your right arm above your head, but be sure not to lock your arm. Count 1 second up and 1 second down. Alternate arms and repeat.

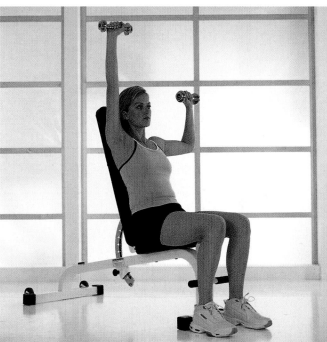

gym: workout 1

step-ups

Go briskly through this exercise: step-ups work your lower body muscles, but they should raise your heart rate, too. Use a step of a suitable height so that your knee does not bend to less than 90 degrees when you step on to it.

Do 25 reps on each side

1 Stand facing a step or stair. Step up with your right foot, placing your whole foot flat on the step. Keep your back straight and your head and neck relaxed.

2 Step up with your left foot so that both feet are flat on the step. Step down one foot at a time, right foot first. Repeat until you've completed a set of reps. As you shape up, this movement will almost be a jog.

gym: workout 1

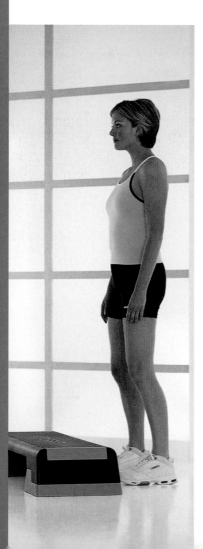
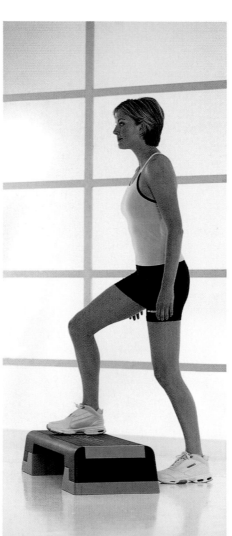
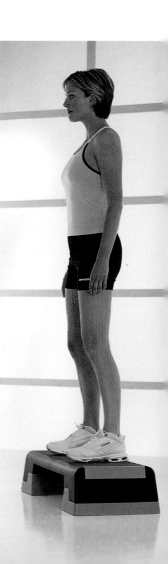

lateral raise (slow)

In the finish position, keep your arms parallel to the floor to ensure that you work all three sections of your shoulder muscles evenly. Take care not to hunch your shoulders—doing so may cause damage to your neck.

Do 15 reps

1 Stand with feet hip-width apart, knees slightly bent. Start with your arms by your sides, holding dumbbells with your palms facing inward. Keep your abdominals tight throughout the exercise.

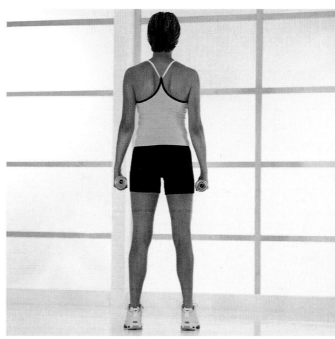

2 Slowly raise your arms away from your sides, keeping your elbows slightly bent, until your hands are at shoulder level. Keep your palms facing downward; don't allow your hands to twist. Keep your torso still. Lower your arms slowly and repeat.

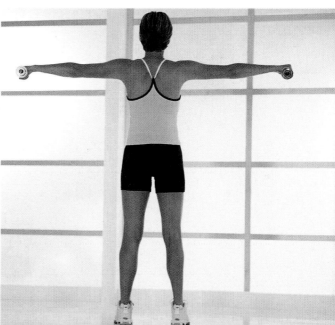

gym: workout 1

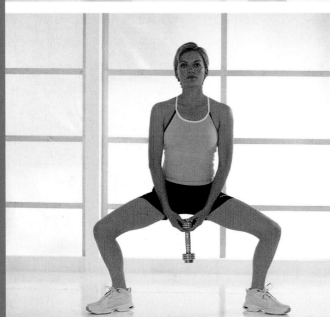

wide leg squat

This is an excellent move to help tone up the backside and inner thighs. It's important to have your knees facing outward at all times, and to keep the movement slow and controlled.

Do 20 reps

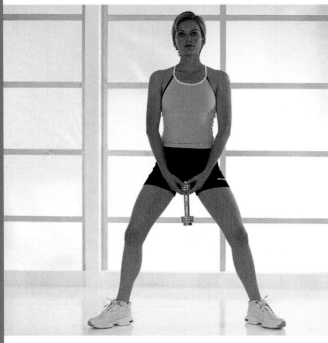

1 Stand with your feet about twice hip-width apart, knees facing outward in a plié-style position. Use a dumbbell to make this exercise slightly more difficult. Hold the dumbbell vertically between your legs.

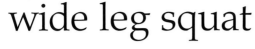

2 Keeping your back straight, bend your knees until your thighs are almost parallel to the floor. Hold for 1 second. Then, keeping your upper body straight, slowly return to the start position.

gym: workout 1

single arm lateral raise

Keep your arm parallel to the floor to ensure that you work all three section of the deltoids, or shoulder muscles, evenly. When doing this exercise, watch yourself in a mirror to check your technique.

Do 15 reps on each side

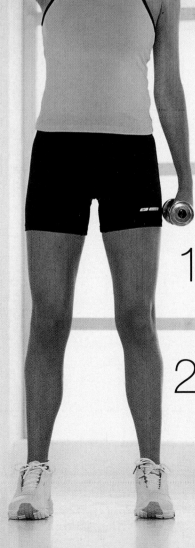

1 Stand with your feet hip-width apart, knees slightly bent. Hold the dumbbells so that your palms face inward.

2 Slowly raise one arm away from your side, your elbow slightly bent, until your hand is at shoulder level. Keep your palm facing down. Keep your torso still. Slowly return to the start position. Complete reps on one arm before switching sides.

gym: workout 1

cross trainer

Before continuing, do a short burst on the cross trainer. This gives your entire body a thorough workout, and will also help to prevent muscles and joints from getting stiff or sore. Stand straight, abdominals pulled in and your feet firmly on the pedals.

Set the cross trainer for 3 min

1 Stand firmly on the pedals and program in the required information, including your height and weight.

2 Gripping the handles, begin by moving your feet forward and backward. Keep the pressure on your legs even. Stand up straight and keep your stomach flat and rear end tucked in.

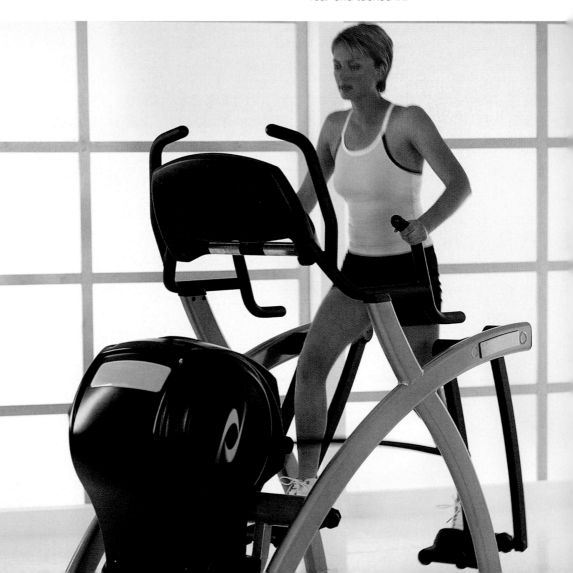

gym: workout 1

What next?

Repeat all exercises starting from the staright arm pulldowns (page 41). Then turn to pages 156–157 and do the full body stretch (the upper body stretch is shown here).

Moving forward

• As you get stronger, you can repeat this routine three times. This will work your muscles harder and stop them from becoming complacent.

• Increase the effectiveness of the step-ups by adding 11lb (5kg) dumbbells.

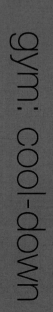

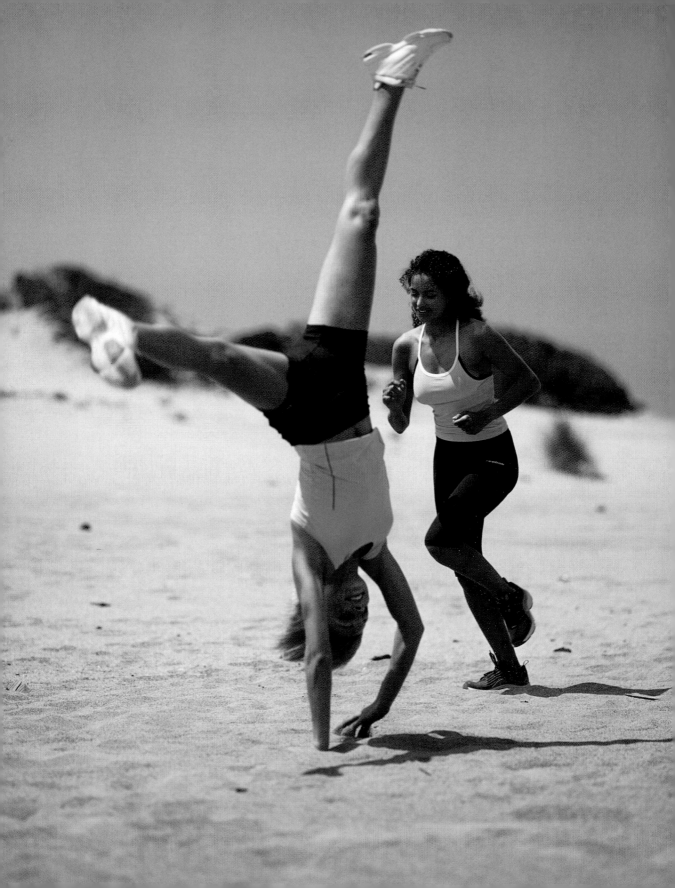

upper body workout 2

This program works the upper body of tube and pear body shapes. Our aim is to strengthen and tone the chest and arms, which will balance out the hips and thighs.

This exercise program is designed to help balance the pear body shape, while providing shape to the straight-up-and-down tube figure. By enhancing the arms, chest and upper back, we'll help to create an illusion of width in the upper body. Pear shapes in particular benefit from this rebalancing; strengthening and visually widening the shoulders and chest area will even out the overall shape. If you are a pear shape, you will soon see that your hips will appear smaller, and your overall posture will dramatically improve, too. The tube shape, on the other hand, benefits from this workout for entirely different reasons. By focusing on the upper body, we will create definition and curves in the upper back and arms. Tube shapes usually have relatively shapeless arms. With this workout, their arms will be as enviable as their legs.

gym: workout 2

exercise	perform	exercise	perform
rower	⅖ mile (700m)	triceps dip	20 reps
seated row	15 reps	bridge	30 secs
lat pulldown	15 reps	alternating biceps curls	30 reps
seated row	12 reps	oblique crunch	20 reps
seated lateral raise	15 reps	lifted knee oblique crunch	20 reps
medicine ball push-up	30 reps	*repeat the workout three times from*	
triceps pushdown	15 reps	*the seated row*	
single arm shoulder press	20 reps per side	*cool-down stretches as prescribed*	

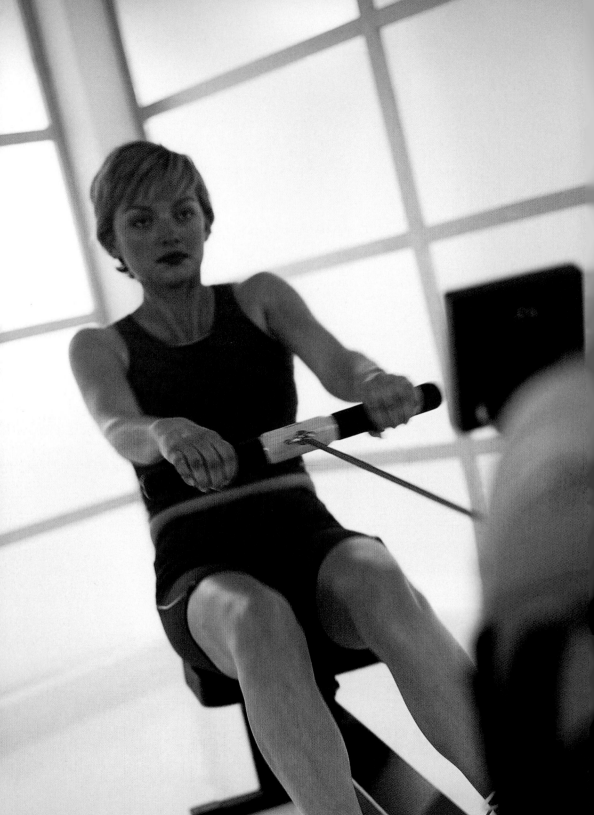

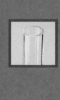

rower

Using a rowing machine provides high-intensity resistance, helping to raise your heart rate and burn large numbers of calories. Rowing is an ideal warm-up, as your entire body is stretched and awakened during the exercise.

Do ⅖ mile (700m) at a steady pace

1 Your legs should be bent, with the knees tucked in close to the chest. Your arms should be straight, extended directly in front of you at shoulder level, and you should have a firm grip on the handles, with your hands positioned directly above your toes. Your torso should tilt forward slightly while your back is held firm.

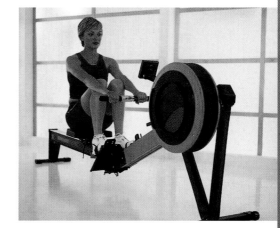

2 Start the first stroke by straightening your legs, using your leg muscles to power the movement and keeping your arms extended in front of you. Keep your torso in the catch position as you start to pull back. Keep your arms straight until they reach your knees, then lean back slightly, pulling the handle toward your chest.

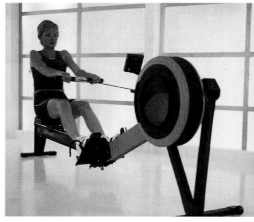

3 Pull your shoulders back so your elbows bend just behind your your body. Your legs should be straight and your body tilted back slightly. As you return to the start position, stretch your arms forward and straighten them as you tilt your body forward, pivoting off the hips. As you slide forward, bend your legs and tuck your knees up close to your chest.

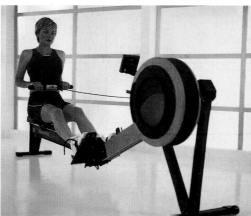

gym: warm-up 2

seated row

This exercise tones the muscles of the upper middle back. To get the most from this move, keep the torso and legs completely still. Working on your back muscles helps build core strength, and goes a long way toward improving your posture.

Do 15 reps

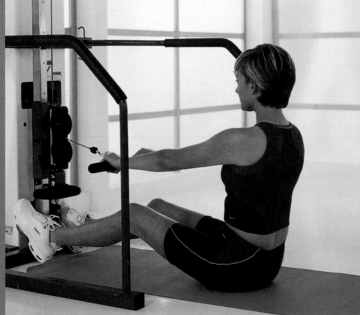

1 Sit on the floor facing the cable machine, legs out in front of you and knees slightly bent. Hold the bar with both hands; take care to keep your back straight.

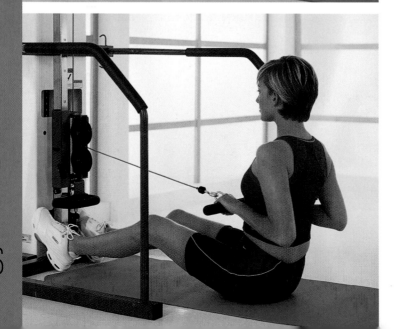

2 Pull the bar in close to your body, aiming for the lower chest area. Hold for 1 second, then return to the start position. Keep your elbows tucked in close to your body.

gym: workout 2

lat pulldown

This exercise works the large muscles of the back—the latissimus dorsi, or lats, and the rhomboids. Pull the bar down for the count of two seconds and raise it, counting to two. Keep your back straight and your abdominals tight at all times.

Do 15 reps

1 Hold the bar firmly with both hands placed slightly more than shoulder-width apart. Keep your feet planted firmly on the floor.

2 Pull down and, as you do so, breathe out. Breathe in as you return to the start position. A single rep should take about 4 seconds.

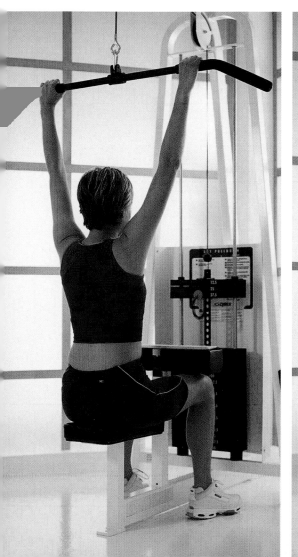

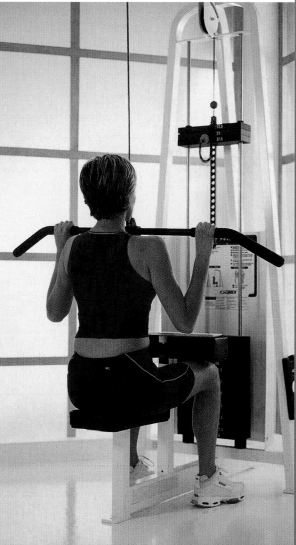

gym: workout 2

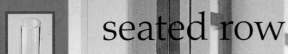

seated row

The seated row (see also page 62) is repeated here because it is such a good exercise for the upper middle back. Keep your elbows tucked in to your sides. This will help to keep your back straight and strong.

Do 12 reps

1 Sit on the floor facing the cable machine, legs out in front of you and knees slightly bent. Hold the bar with both hands; take care to keep your back straight.

2 Pull the bar in close to the body, aiming for the lower chest area. Hold for 1 second, then return to the start position. Repeat until you have completed the required number of reps.

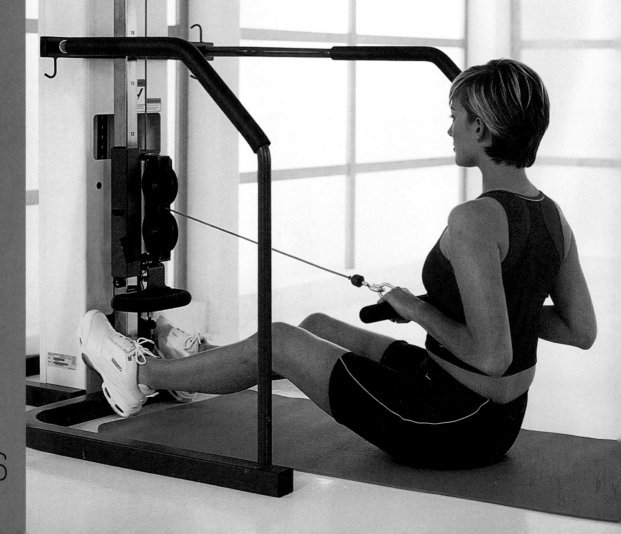

gym: workout 2

seated lateral raise

When performing this exercise, keep your arms strong and steady. This ensures you have worked all three sections of the shoulder muscles evenly. Using a seat or bench for the exercise helps to support your lower back.

Do 15 reps

1 Sit on a bench with your back flat against the support. Grasp the dumbbells firmly, keeping your arms parallel to the floor. Your arms should be slightly bent, and your hands turned slightly in. Raise your arms very slowly, taking care to not tense your neck.

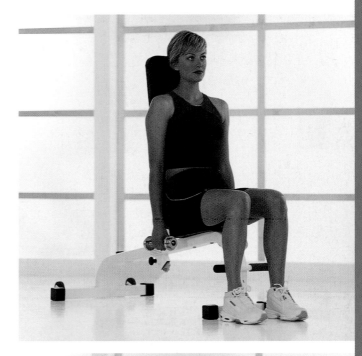

2 When the dumbbells reach shoulder level, your arms should be parallel to the floor. Pause at this point for a second, while keeping your thumbs turned slightly down. Lower the dumbbells very slowly, keeping your arms slightly bent. Lower the dumbbell to a point just slightly away from the body and complete the required number of reps.

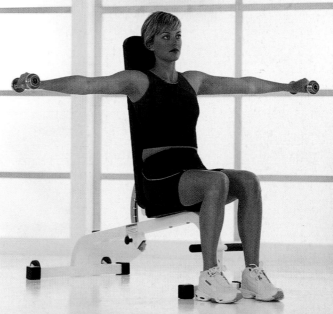

gym: workout 2

medicine ball push-up

This exercise uses a medicine ball instead of dumbbells. This allows the effort required to be evenly distributed through your body. Remember to keep your back straight and strong, and take care not to tip your hips forward.

Do 30 reps

1 Stand with feet shoulder-width apart, knees relaxed. Hold the medicine ball in front of your face, slightly lowered.

2 Gripping the ball, stretch your arms above your head, keeping your lower body still. Return to the start position, and repeat.

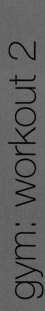

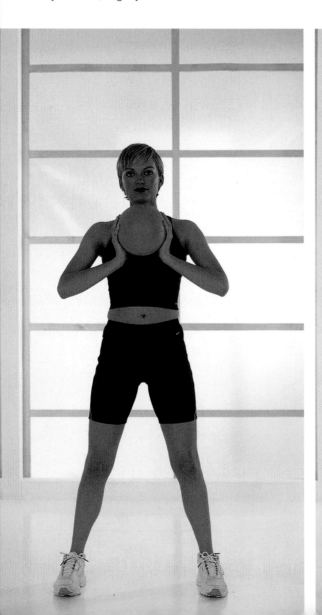

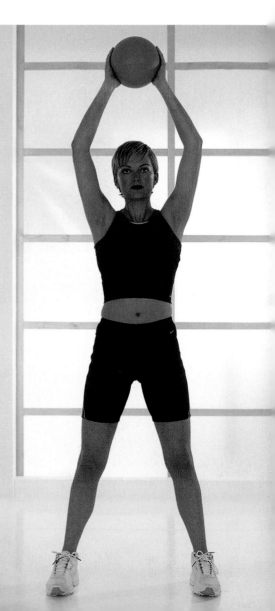

gym: workout 2

triceps pushdown

To achieve optimum results from this exercise, keep your hands close together. This works the biceps and lat muscles. This exercise is quite advanced—use control to complete it, rather than momentum.

Do 15 reps

1 Stand upright facing the cable tower. Grip the bar with the palms facing down and about 10–12in (25–30cm) apart.

2 Push the bar down to the front of your thighs. Pause and raise slowly to the start. Keep your elbows close to your sides.

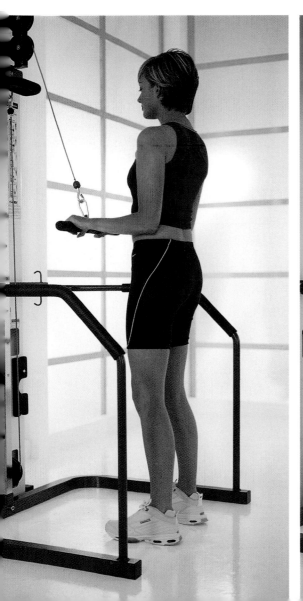

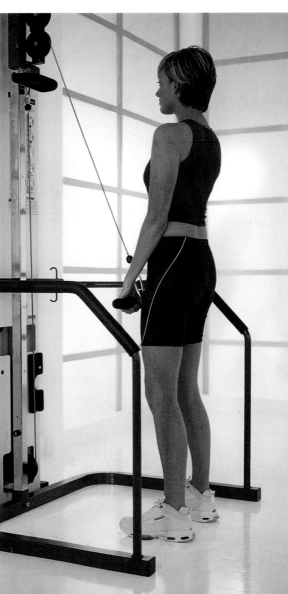

gym: workout 2

ngle arm shoulder press

xercise works the deltoids, or shoulder muscles, helping to create depth and width in the upper body. Working the arms, shoulders, and chest area will help to balance out the lower body, making hips and thighs appear smaller.

Do 20 reps on each side

1 Sit with your back well supported by the bench and legs bent at about 90°. Hold a dumbbell in each hand with your arms bent at 90° and elbows out at shoulder level.

2 Press the dumbbell upward, raising your arm above your head, but be sure not to lock your arm straight. Your body should not move. Count 1 second up and 1 second down. Repeat, then change sides.

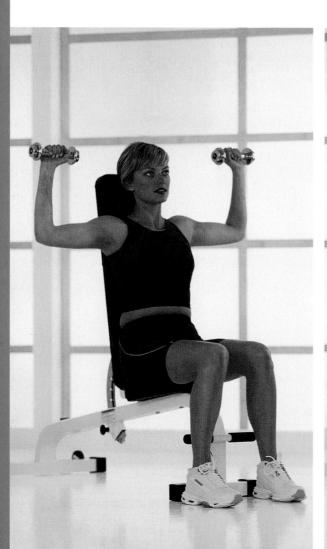

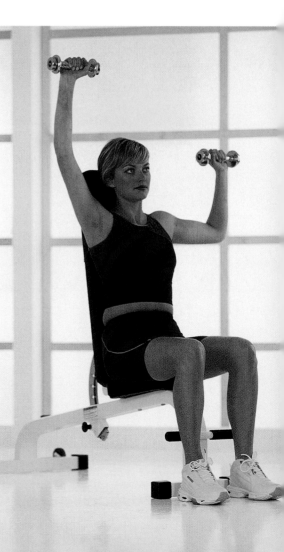

triceps dip

Your triceps are the muscles at the backs of your arms, and are generally one of the first areas to become flabby and untoned. The triceps dip is extremely effective for strengthening and toning this area. Don't lock your arms, and take it slowly.

Do 20 reps, increasing to 30 reps with practice

1 Sitting with your back to a bench, position your heels 2–3ft (60–90cm) in front of you. Grip the edge of the bench with an overhand wide grip (palms facing the bench) and push yourself up so that your arms are fully extended and perpendicular to the floor.

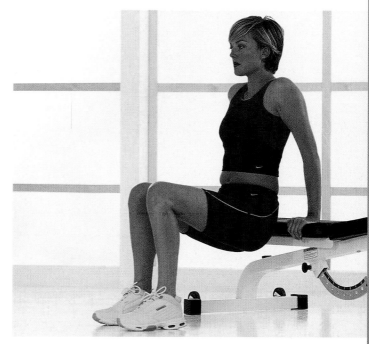

2 Bending your arms, descend toward the floor until your upper arms are parallel to the floor. Push back up to the starting position. As you get stronger, and the exercise gets easier, move your feet farther away from the bench. Always keep your back close to the bench.

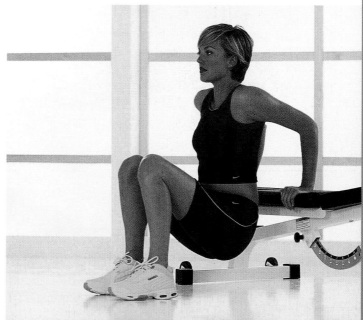

gym: workout 2

bridge

This is a relatively advanced exercise and proof that you don't always have to move your muscles in order to strengthen them. Start slowly and work your way up to a more advanced level.

Hold for 30 seconds, increasing to 45 seconds with practice

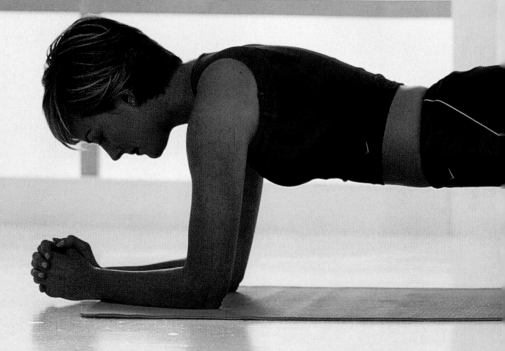

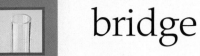

gym: workout 2

Position yourself so that your toes are on the ground and your elbows are directly below your shoulders. Raise yourself up, keeping a straight line from your shoulders to your ankles, so that your elbows and toes support your body. Use your abdominals to maintain the position, and take care not to stick your backside up in the air. Repeat the hold. This exercise works your abdominal muscles hard, so take your time perfecting it.

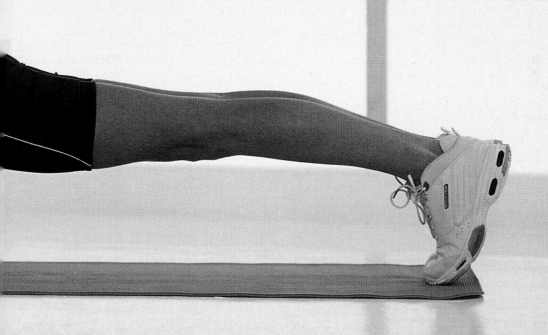

gym: workout 2

lternating biceps curls

This is a great "isolating" exercise. Focusing on the biceps gives fantastic definition to the upper arm, which can be a problem area for many women, especially as they get older. Well-defined arms immediately enhance the appearance of the upper body.

Do 30 reps

1 Stand with your feet hip-width apart, knees slightly bent, and your arms by your sides. Turn your arms out and hold the dumbbells so that your palms face forward.

2 Bend either arm alternately to lift the dumbbell toward your shoulders. Keep your elbows tucked in close to your body. At the top, flex your biceps to maximize the effectiveness of the exercise.

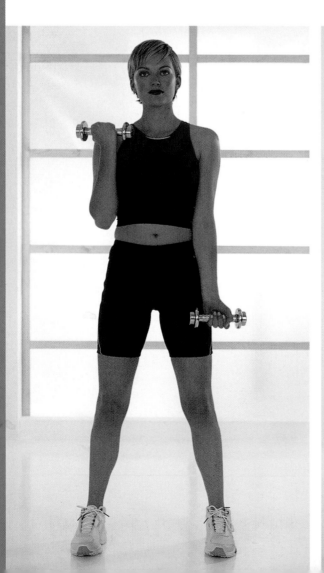
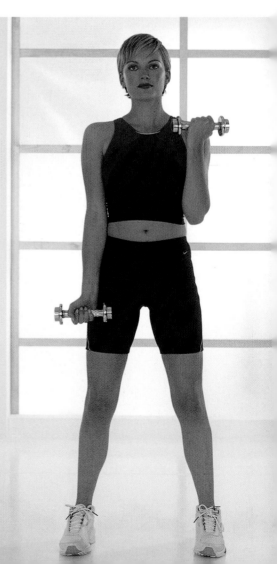

gym: workout 2

oblique crunch

Working the obliques—the muscles at the side of the stomach that run from under the rib cage to the hips—will help tone and minimize this area. This helps to give the illusion of a V-shaped figure.

Do 20 reps on each side, increasing to 30 reps

1 Lie on your back on a mat with your knees bent, feet flat on the floor, and hands on either side of your head.

2 Slowly raise one shoulder and elbow up toward the outside of the opposite thigh. When you've completed the reps, change shoulders to work the muscles on the other side.

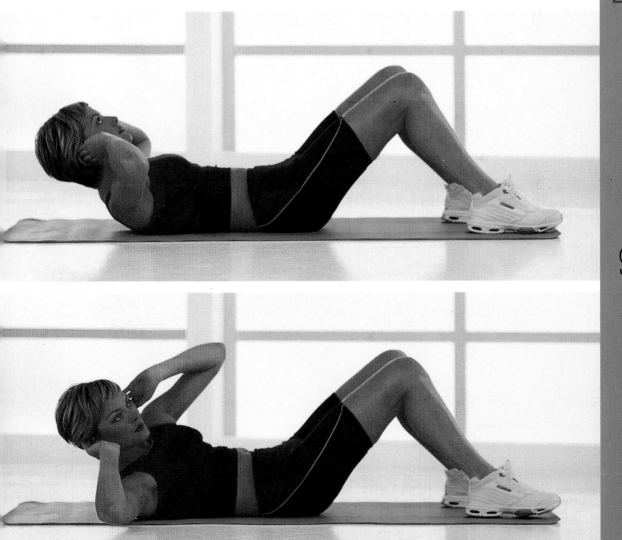

gym: workout 2

lifted knee oblique crunch

Raising your knee in the air for this exercise means you use your abdominal muscles to keep your balance. Make sure you keep your raised knee still to maximize the toning and strengthening benefits of the exercise.

Do 20 reps on each side, increasing to 30 reps

1 Lie on your back with your legs on the ground. Raise your right knee so that your knee and thigh are at 90° to the floor. Keep your stomach muscles pulled in tight and your back pressed into the floor.

2 Raise your left elbow and shoulder toward your right knee. Return to the start position. Repeat until you have completed all the crunches on one side, then switch to the other side.

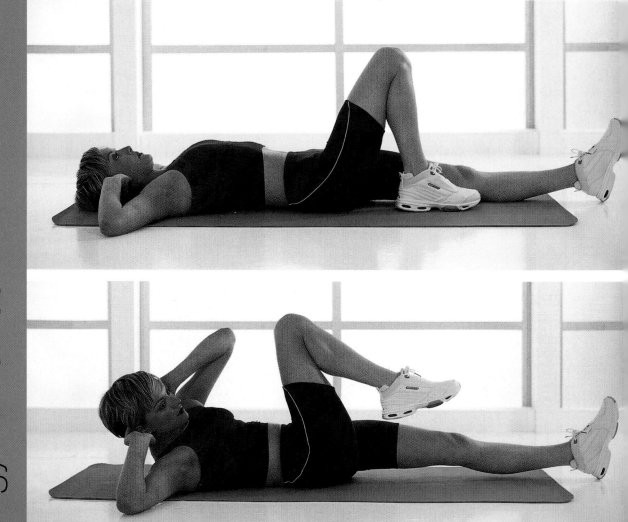

gym: workout 2

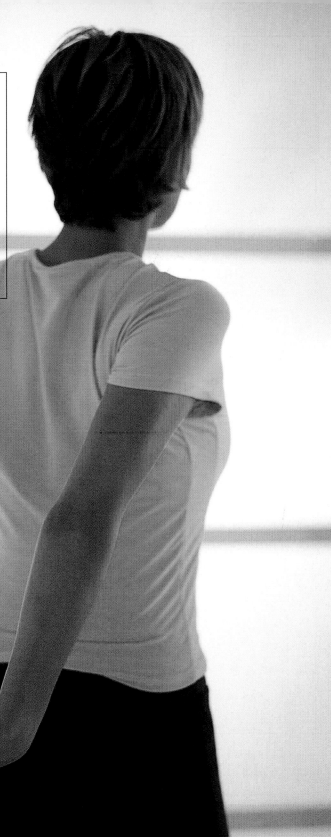

What next?

Repeat the workout, from the seated row (page 62), two more times. Then turn to pages 156–157 and do the full body stretch (the chest stretch is shown here).

Moving forward

As you get stronger, you can do the workout four times.

Over a period of time, increase your rowing distance to ½ mile (750m).).

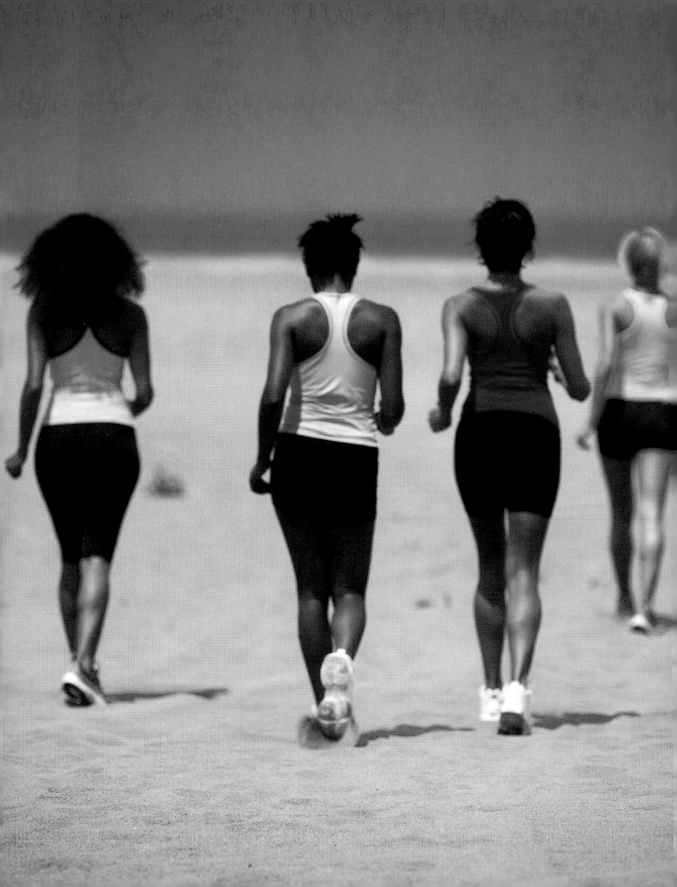

total body workout 3

This workout is designed for all body shapes. Whether you're a pear, tube, apple, or hourglass shape, you'll tone and strengthen your entire body without gaining any mass.

This program involves working on gym machines to do high-repetition exercises with moderate resistance. This helps to condition the entire body by burning fat effectively and boosting your metabolism (the rate at which you burn calories). Not only will your body look and feel stronger, but your limbs will look and feel leaner, and you'll find that as you increase the level of resistance and number of repetitions, your level of fitness will also improve. When you are training, make sure that you choose machine settings that challenge your fitness levels for the last 4–5 repetitions and exhaust your body.

gym: workout 3

exercise	perform	exercise	perform
cross trainer	6 min	wide leg squat	25 reps
lat pulldown	25 reps	seated leg curl	20 reps
chest press	20 reps	wall position biceps curls	20 reps
walking lunge	20 reps	fitness ball squats	30 reps
alternating squat thrusts	40 reps	crunch	20 reps
push-ups	25 reps	reverse curl	25 reps
fast step-ups	40 reps per leg	oblique knee pull (alternate)	30 reps
seated row	25 reps	*repeat the workout from the lat pulldown*	
tricep dips	20 reps	*cool-down stretches as prescribed*	
bench step-overs	50 reps		

cross trainer

Even if you're quite fit, you should always warm up before an exercise program to avoid damaging muscles and ligaments. Don't overdo it—a warm-up should be a gentle introduction to the workout ahead.

Do 6 minutes

1 Stand firmly on the pedals and program in the required information. Set the machine for 6 minutes and the MHR to 75%.

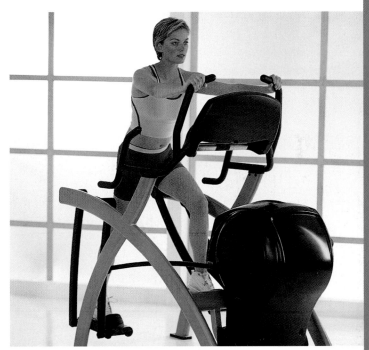

2 Gripping the handles, begin by pushing your feet forward. Remember to keep the pressure on your legs even. Stand up straight and keep your stomach flat and rear end tucked in.

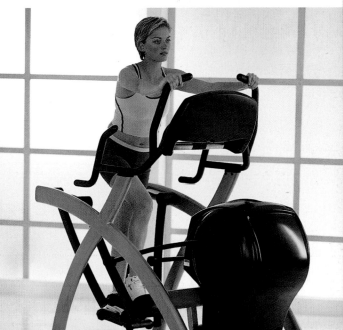

gym: warm-up 3

lat pulldown

This exercise works the large muscles of the back—the latissimus dorsi, or lats, and the rhomboids. As well as the toning effect, strengthening your back will help prevent back problems later in life.

Do 25 reps

1 Hold the bar firmly with both hands placed slightly wider than shoulder-width apart. Keep your back straight and your abdominals tight at all times.

2 Pull down and, as you do so, breathe out for the count of two. Breathe in to the count of two and return to the start position. Rest for a moment and repeat.

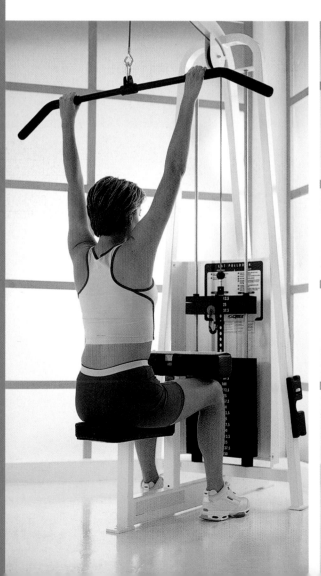

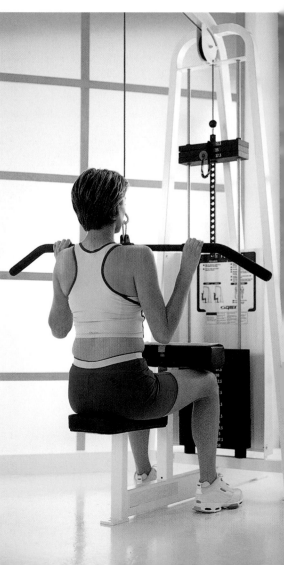

gym: workout 3

chest press

The chest press machine is a standard piece of equipment in many gyms and is great for building strength and shape into the chest area and triceps (the muscle at the back of the upper arm).

Do 20 reps

1 Ensure that your lower back is supported by the machine. Start with your arms bent at 90°, making sure your elbows are held between chest and shoulder height. Push forward until your arms are almost straight.

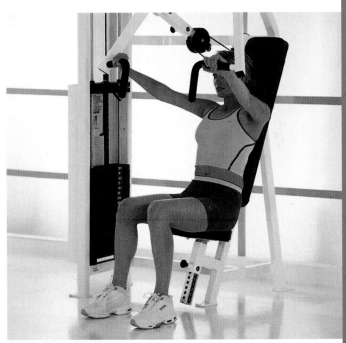

2 Now pull your arms back until your elbows are level with your shoulders. Keep the movement slow and controlled. Count to 2 on the out movement and again to 2 on the inward movement to ensure you are not rushing.

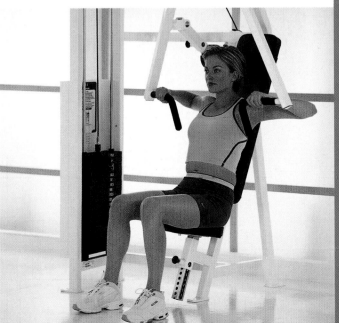

gym: workout 3

walking lunge

Unlike repetitive exercises that often focus on very specific sets of muscles, the continuous forward movement of the walking lunge ensures that all the muscles of your legs and midsection work hard.

Do 20 lunges

1 Stand with feet hip-width apart, knees slightly bent and hands relaxed by your sides. Look straight ahead at a fixed point. This will help you keep your balance.

2 Step forward so that your foot is about one stride-length from your back foot. As you do this, lower your body, then hold the position for 1 second.

gym: workout 3

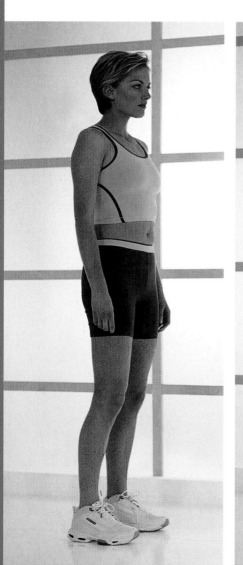
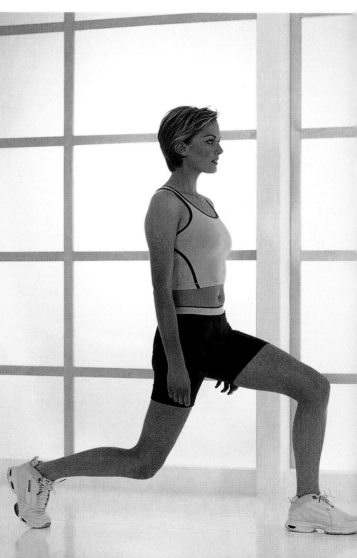

"Using the resistance of your own body weight is a simple way to tone, strengthen, and shape up. It's quick and effective—and you don't need any special equipment."

3 Raise your body, lifting your back leg as you do so; then, keeping your body straight and strong, begin to move your back foot forward to repeat the lunge with that leg.

4 Step forward another stride-length. Repeat the movement of lowering your body down, and hold again for 1 second. Repeat the required number of lunges, switching direction whenever you need to.

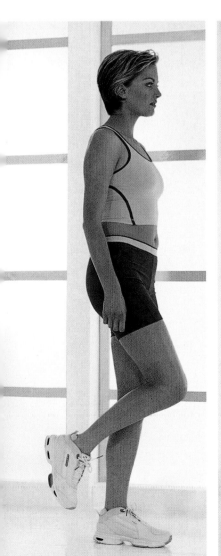

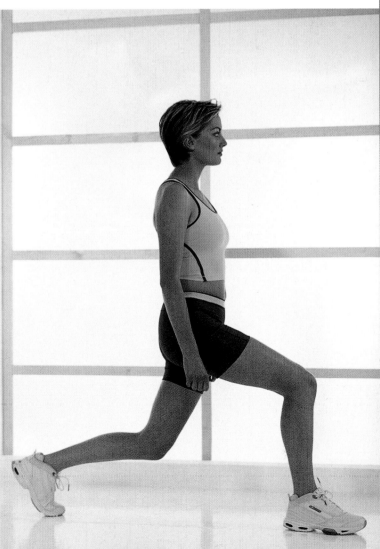

gym: workout 3

alternating squat thrusts

Keep your back steady and strong throughout this movement. To work your legs and abdominals even harder, stretch your legs out as far as possible. Make sure your neck is relaxed and in line with your spine. Keep your eyes focused on the mat.

Do 40 reps

gym: workout 3

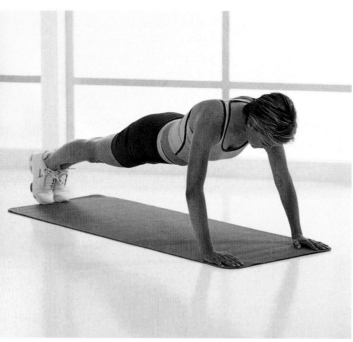

1 Position yourself as though you're about to complete a push-up. Your arms should be slightly wider than shoulder-width apart. Pick a spot on the mat and keep your eyes fixed to it. This way you won't lift your neck, or lose your balance.

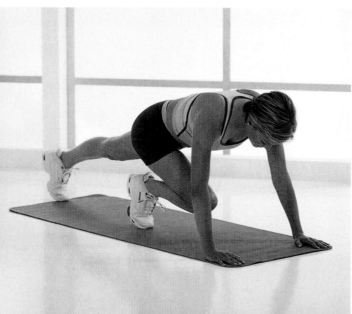

2 Bring your right knee forward until it almost meets the right elbow. The left leg remains extended. Immediately return the right leg to the start position, and bring the left knee forward. The movements are alternating and continuous. You can do this exercise quickly, but keep your movements steady.

push-ups

The push-up uses the weight of the body to work the triceps, pectorals,, and deltoids (arm, chest, and shoulder muscles). Start with the half push-up and progress to the full push-up once you have built up strength.

Do 25 reps

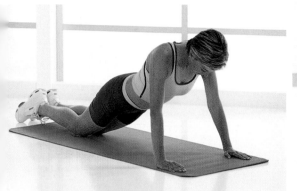

1 Place your hands directly under your shoulders with your fingers pointing forward. Keep your torso and legs straight. If you're doing a half push-up, then bend your knees slightly, as shown. Otherwise, use the start position in step 1 opposite.

2 Bend your arms to about 90° and slowly lower your body almost down to the mat, keeping your head down and neck relaxed. Tighten your stomach and thigh muscles; this will help to keep your legs straight. Be careful not to point your rear end up in the air. Push yourself back up to the start position and repeat.

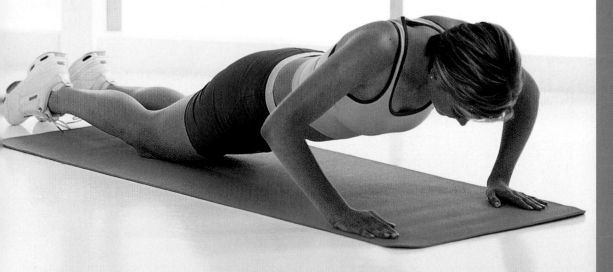

gym: workout 3

fast step-ups

Do this exercise as briskly as you can: step-ups work your lower body muscles but they should also raise your heart rate, thereby burning fat and calories. The harder you work, the quicker you'll achieve a slimmer, more toned silhouette.

Do 40 step-ups on each leg

1 Adjust the step so that your knee does not bend to less than 90° when you step onto it. Step up with one foot, placing your foot flat on the step. Keep your back straight and your head and neck relaxed.

2 Step up with your other foot so that both feet are flat on the step. Step down with your leading foot: land on your toes, then roll the foot down until the heel touches the floor. Repeat, alternating the leading foot.

gym: workout 3

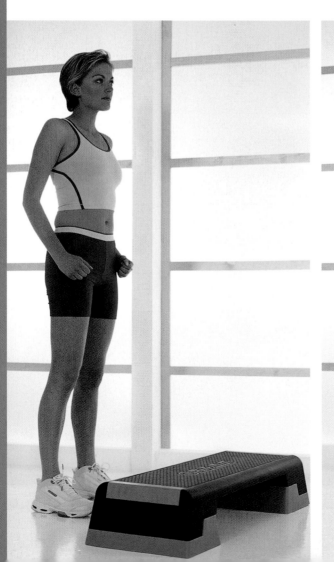

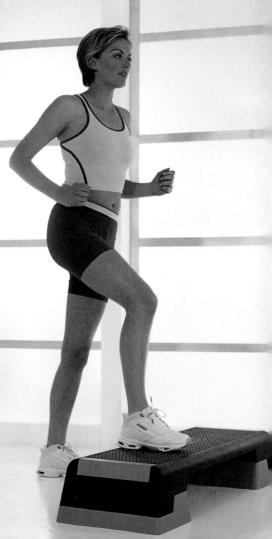

seated row

This exercise tones the muscles of the upper middle back and strengthens the abdominals. To get the most from this exercise, keep the torso and legs completely still. Strong stomach muscles provide stability and strength for your whole body.

Do 25 reps

1 Sit on the floor facing the cable machine, legs out in front of you and knees slightly bent. Hold the bar with both hands, taking care to keep your back straight and firm.

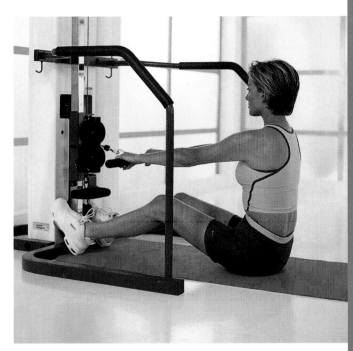

2 Pull the bar in close to your body, aiming for the lower chest area. Hold for 1 second, then return to the starting position. Keep your elbows tucked in close to your body, your stomach pulled in tight.

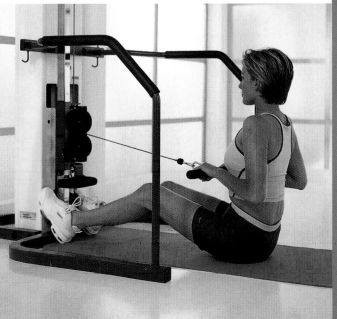

gym: workout 3

triceps dips

This upper-arm exercise tones and strengthens the backs of the arms, which are often prone to flabbiness. Start slowly, working your way up to the higher number of reps as your strength and fitness levels increase.

Do 20 reps, increasing to 30 reps

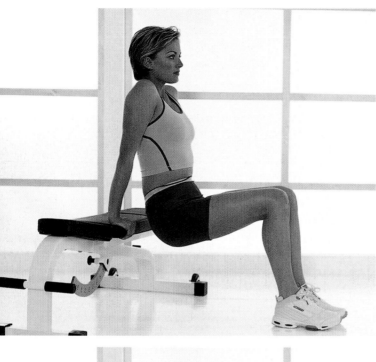

1 Sitting with your back to a bench, position your heels 2–3ft (60–90cm) in front of you. Grip the edge of the bench with an overhand wide grip (palms facing the bench) and push yourself up so that your arms are fully extended and perpendicular to the floor.

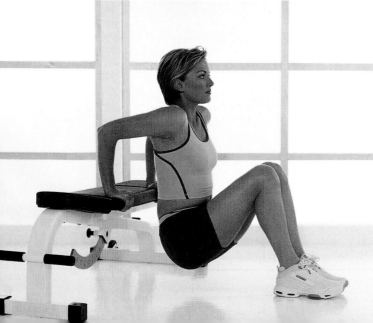

2 Bending your arms, descend toward the floor until your upper arms are parallel to the floor. Push back up to the starting position. As you get stronger, and the exercise gets easier, move your feet farther away from the bench. Always keep your back close to the bench.

gym: workout 3

bench step-overs

By using your body as the weight, this resistance exercise strengthens and tones the legs. Make sure your knee does not bend to less than 90 degrees when you step onto the bench. Fix your eyes on a point in front of you to help you keep your balance.

Do 50 reps

1 Stand sideways to a bench with your arms loosely by your sides. Place one foot on the bench. Use that leg to pull yourself onto the bench so that you are standing upright, facing forward.

2 Transfer your body weight onto the other leg, and slowly lower the opposite leg down onto the floor. When that foot touches the floor, pull yourself back onto the bench and repeat.

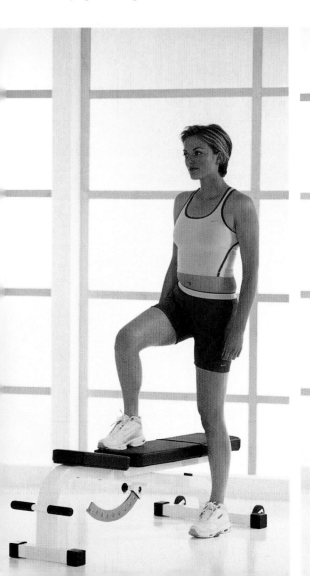

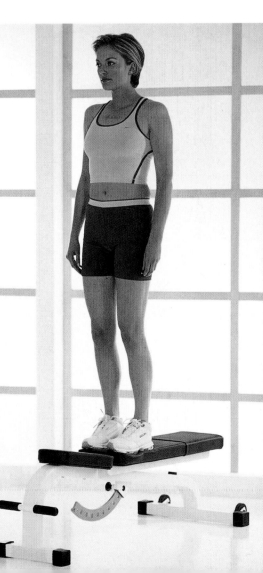

gym: workout 3

ide leg squat

work your inner thighs and tone your backside with this move. Keep your upper body straight, taking care not to bend forward. To make this move harder, use a dumbbell weighing at least 11lb (5kg).

Do 25 reps

1 Stand with your feet about twice hip-width apart, knees facing outward as shown. Hold the dumbbell vertically between your legs. This will help steady the movement.

2 Bend your knees until your thighs are almost parallel to the floor. Hold for 1 second. Then, keeping your upper body straight, slowly return to the start position.

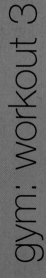

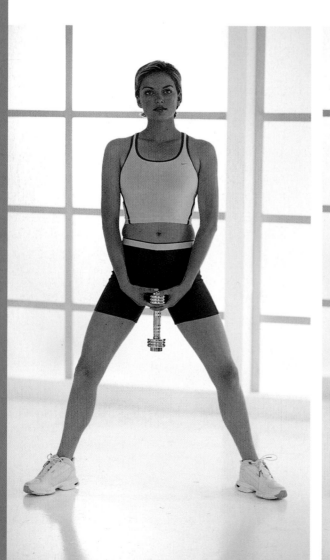

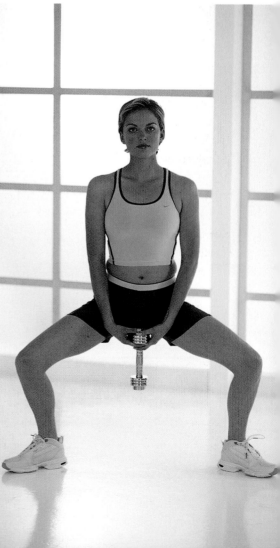

gym: workout 3

seated leg curl

This machine, the leg extension, works the hamstrings—the large muscles at the backs of the thighs. Your reward is longer-looking legs and a slimmer rear end. As the muscles develop, they can also increase your body's calorie-burning potential.

Do 20 reps

1 Sit with your legs extended and your ankles on top of the roller pad. Your back should be at right angles to your legs and your lower back should be supported throughout the exercise. Aim to spread the movement over 6 seconds: 3 seconds to bend the legs and 3 seconds to extend them.

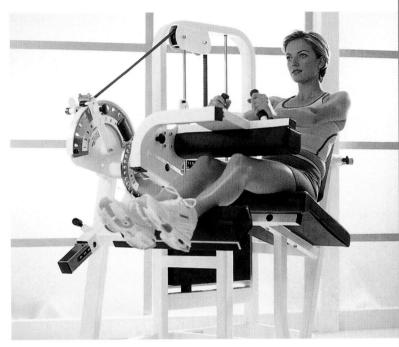

2 Hold your stomach tight and bend your legs, bringing your heels toward your bottom. Hold for 1 second, then slowly return to the start position. Exhale as you lift the weights and inhale as you lower them.

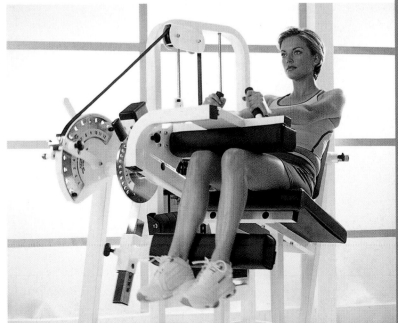

gym: workout 3

wall position biceps curls

This is an exceptionally good and intensive exercise for creating definition and strength in the biceps—the ideal way to tone your upper arms.

Do 20 reps

1 Stand with your back against a wall, feet slightly apart, and arms by your sides. Hold a dumbbell in each hand, with the weights parallel to the floor.

2 Keeping your elbows pressed firmly against the wall, raise your forearms toward your shoulders. Hold for 1 second, then lower. Breathe deeply and evenly, keeping the movements as controlled as possible.

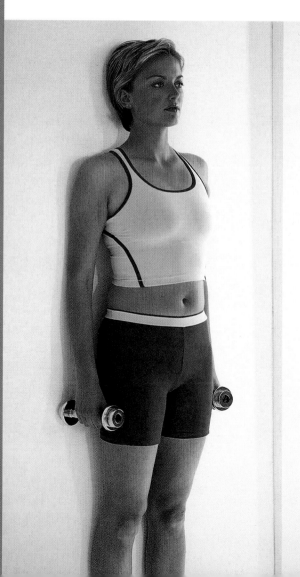
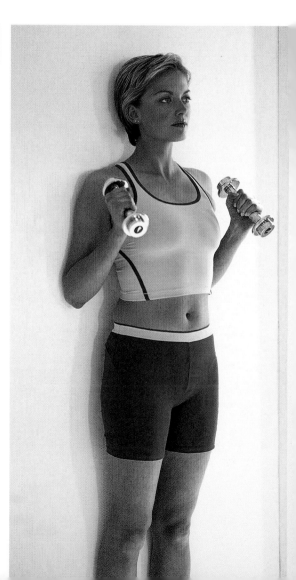

gym: workout 3

fitness ball squats

Using a fitness ball for these squats allows you to put your body weight farther back toward your heels, and increases pressure on the buttocks and inner thighs.

Do 30 reps

1 Position a fitness ball between the wall and your lower and middle back. Keep your back upright and straight, your tummy in, and your knees slightly bent. Relax your hands and arms.

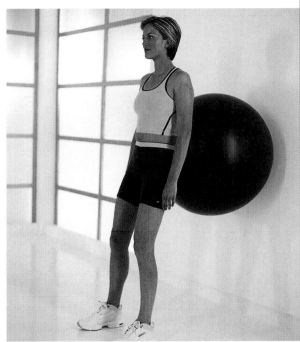

2 Slowly lower your body down until your thighs are parallel to the floor. While doing this exercise, make sure your back is straight and the full pressure of your body weight is placed against the ball. Slowly push yourself back to the starting position. You can make the exercise work harder for you by squeezing your buttocks on the way down and on the way up, and by moving your feet farther away from the wall.

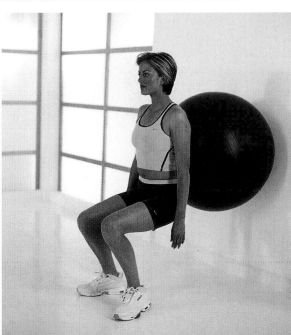

gym: workout 3

crunch

Tone your tummy with simple sit-ups or crunches. You don't have to do hundreds a day to achieve a flat stomach, just make sure you do them properly. A well-defined waist creates an illusion of curves, balancing the upper and lower areas.

Do 20 reps, increasing to 30 reps

1 Lie on your back with your legs hip-width apart, knees bent. Place your hands by your ears. Breathe in, and tighten your stomach muscles.

2 On the out breath, raise your shoulders and chest upward, at the same time keeping your neck relaxed and looking up at the ceiling. Lower to the floor and repeat.

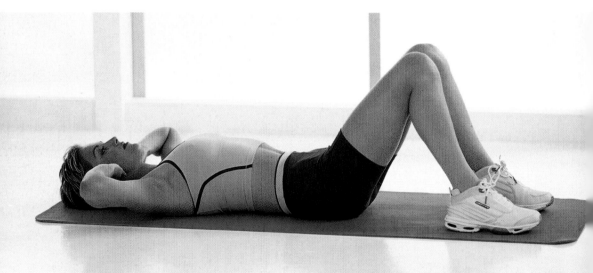

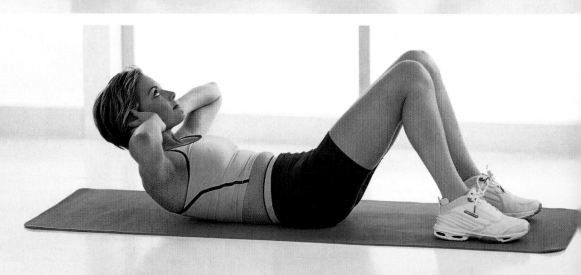

gym: workout 3

reverse curl

Many people find that the reverse curl puts less strain on the neck area than the crunch (see opposite). Make sure you use your stomach muscles to lift your lower abdomen, not the momentum of the exercise.

Do 25 reps, increasing to 30 reps

1 Lie on your back with your arms by your sides, legs at 90° to your body and knees slightly bent. Place your hands by your ears. Keep your shoulders and head on the floor at all times.

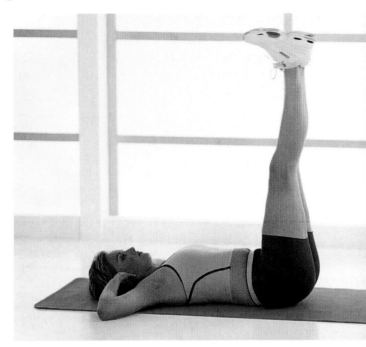

2 Tighten your lower abdominals and curl your legs and pelvis toward your rib cage. Keep your upper legs at 90° to your torso so that the movement is performed by the abdominals rather than the momentum from the legs. As you gain strength, work your way up to the harder set.

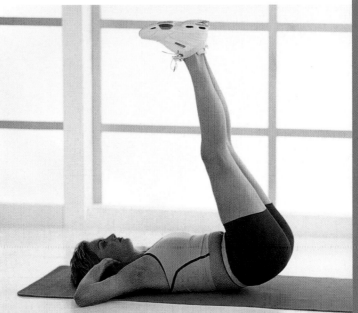

gym: workout 3

oblique knee-pull (alternating)

Aim to get your shoulder as close as possible to your knee. The closer you get, the better the workout is for your waistline. Keep the movements steady and your neck and shoulders relaxed.

Do 30 reps, increasing to 40 reps with practice

1 Lie on your back with one foot flat on the floor and the other leg raised so your thigh is at right angles to the floor. Place your hands by your ears and keep your shoulders down.

2 Pull your belly button toward your spine and raise your right shoulder and elbow toward your left knee. Keep your hips on the floor. Return to the starting position. Repeat for the full set, then switch sides.

gym: workout 3

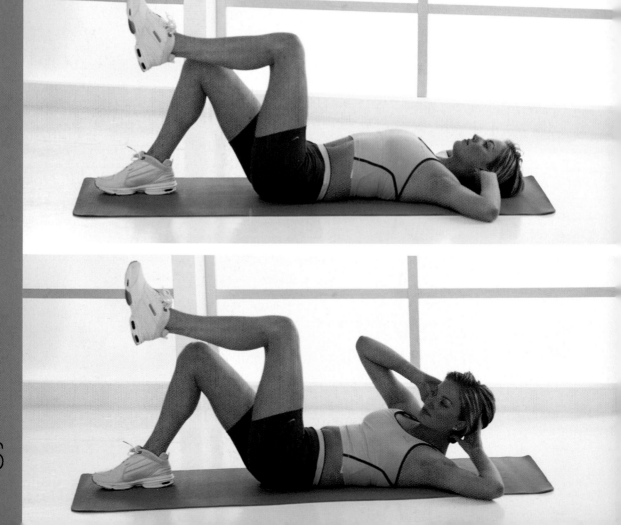

What next?

Repeat the sequence one more time, starting from the chest press (page 81). Once you've repeated all the exercises, turn to pages 156–157 and do the full body stretch (the hamstring stretch is shown here).

Moving forward

• Work on your technique—it's more important than speed.

• Aim to increase your workout to the maximum number of reps within four weeks of beginning the program.

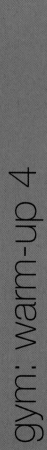

rower

To achieve maximum results from the rowing machine, make sure you are generating the majority of the stroke power with your legs.

Do ⅖ mile (700m) at a steady pace

1 Your legs should be bent, with your knees tucked in close to your chest. Your arms should be straight, extended directly in front of you at shoulder level, and you should have a firm grip on the handles, with your hands positioned directly above your toes. Your torso should tilt forward slightly while your back is held firm.

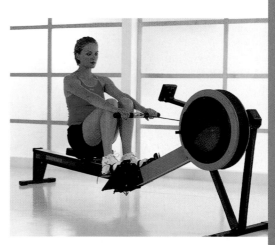

2 Start the first stroke by straightening your legs, using your leg muscles to power the movement. Keep your arms extended in front of you. Your torso should remain in an upright position as you start to pull back. Keep your arms straight until they reach your knees, then lean back slightly, pulling the handle toward your chest.

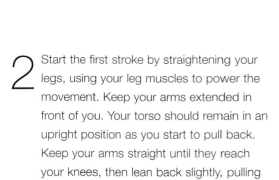

3 Pull your shoulders back so your elbows bend just behind your body. Your legs should be straight and your body tilted back slightly. As you return to the start position, stretch your arms forward and straighten them as you tilt the body forward, pivoting from the hips. As you slide forward, bend your legs and tuck your knees up close to your chest.

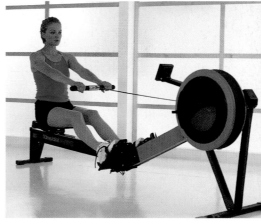

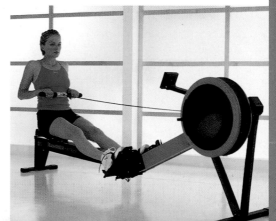

gym: warm-up 4

close grip pulldowns

Performing the pulldowns with a close grip works the biceps and the lat muscles. Keep your movements slow and steady. This ensures that you are performing the exercise correctly and will get the maximum benefit from it.

Do 15 reps, increasing to 20 reps

1 Hold the bar with your hands slightly more than shoulder-width apart, using an underhand grip. Make sure to keep your back straight throughout the exercise.

2 Pull the bar down, until it is at chest level. Keep your body as straight as possible. Hold for 1 second, then slowly return the bar to the start position.

gym: workout 4

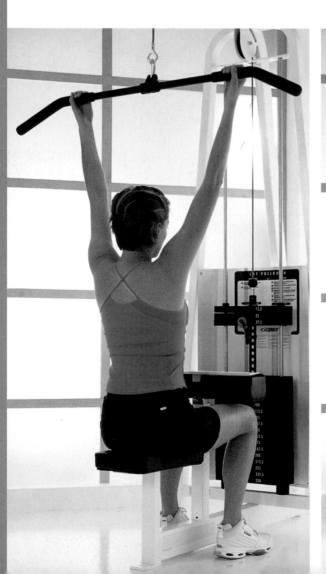

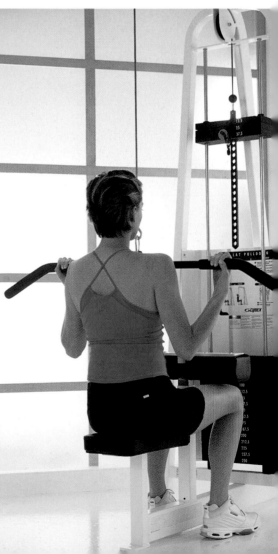

seated row

This exercise tones the muscles of the upper middle back. To get the most from this exercise, keep the torso and legs completely still. The back muscles are often neglected, but they are an integral part of your overall health and fitness.

Do 10 reps, increasing to 12 then 15 reps

1 Sit on the floor facing the cable machine, legs out in front of you and knees slightly bent. Hold the bar with both hands; take care to keep your back straight and still.

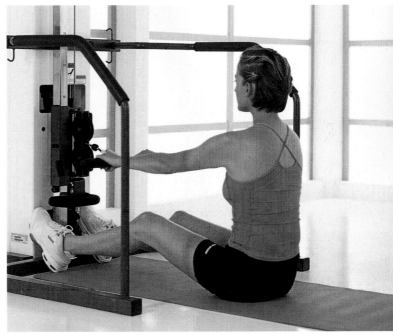

2 Pull the bar in close to your body, aiming for the lower chest area. Hold for 1 second, then return to the start position. Keep your elbows tucked in close to your body.

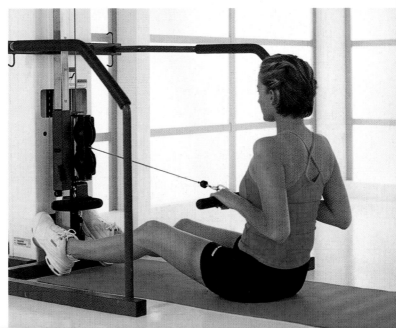

gym: workout 4

reverse fly

This is quite a tough exercise that targets a specific area—the muscles across the back of the shoulders and in the middle of the back. Take care not to curve your back upward when you lift the weights.

Do 15 reps, increasing to 20 reps

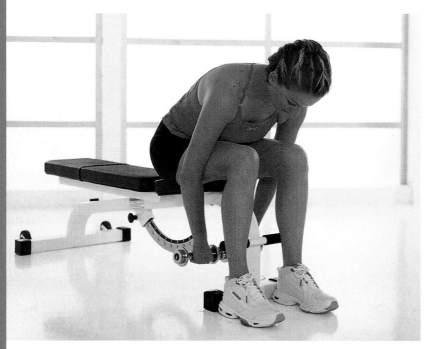

1 Sit on the end of the bench with knees bent at about 90° and feet hip-width apart. Bend forward, keeping your back straight, and start by holding the weights behind your calves, thumbs facing inward.

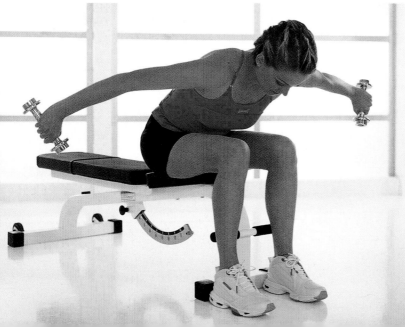

2 Lift the weights, keeping your arms slightly bent, until your elbows are level with your shoulders. Hold for 2 seconds, then slowly return to the start position and repeat.

gym: workout 4

hyperextension

This exercise is an excellent way to strengthen your lower back. Too often, poor posture, especially when sitting at a desk, can lead to weak and underdeveloped lower back muscles.

Do 20 reps, increasing to 25 then 30 reps

Lie down flat on your front on the floor. Tuck your elbows in close to your body. Keeping your hips on the floor, push your torso up until you are supporting your body weight on your elbows. Be careful to keep your neck relaxed. Hold for 15 seconds. Return to the starting position.

Rest for 2 minutes. Repeat the last four exercises, then move on. As you increase the number of reps, rest for 1–1½ minutes before repeating the last four exercises 2 to 4 times. Then move on to the next group of exercises.

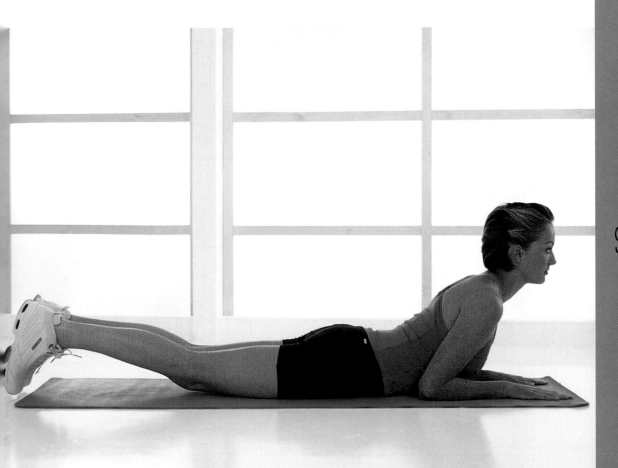

gym: workout 4

upright row

This is a good exercise for the shoulder muscles and the biceps, the muscles at the front of the upper arms. Choose your dumbbells according to your fitness level: start with 11lb (5kg) dumbbells and gradually increase the weight.

Do 15 reps, increasing to 20 reps

1 Stand with your feet hip-width apart, legs slightly bent and back straight. Hold the weights in front of you so that your palms face your thighs.

2 Pull the weights up to chest height, leading with the elbows. Slowly lower the weights and return to the start position. Count 2 seconds up and 2 seconds down.

gym: workout 4

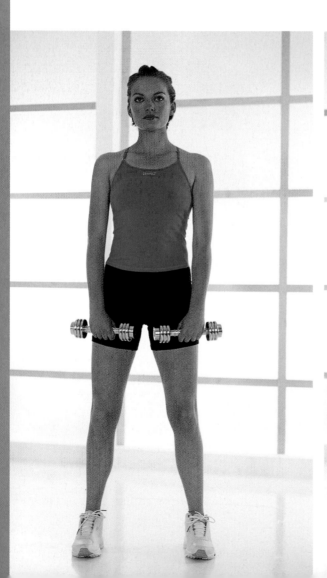
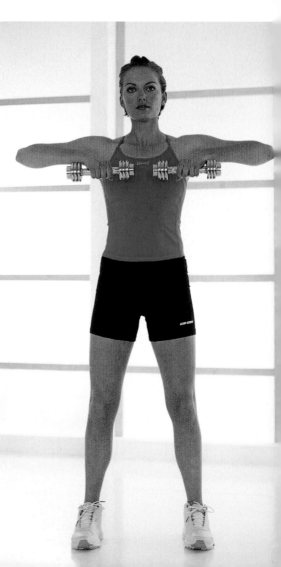

lateral raise

Keep your arms parallel to the floor when they are raised, to ensure that you work all three sections of the deltoids, or shoulder muscles, evenly.

Do 10 reps, increasing to 12 then 15 reps

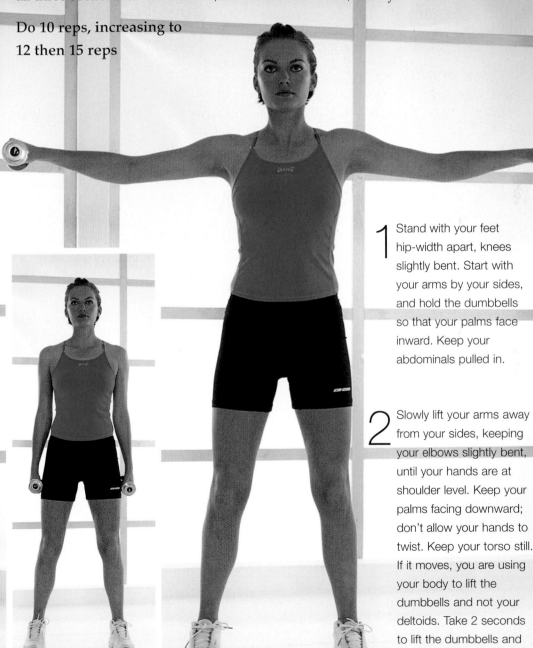

1 Stand with your feet hip-width apart, knees slightly bent. Start with your arms by your sides, and hold the dumbbells so that your palms face inward. Keep your abdominals pulled in.

2 Slowly lift your arms away from your sides, keeping your elbows slightly bent, until your hands are at shoulder level. Keep your palms facing downward; don't allow your hands to twist. Keep your torso still. If it moves, you are using your body to lift the dumbbells and not your deltoids. Take 2 seconds to lift the dumbbells and 2 seconds to lower them.

gym: workout 4

single arm raises

This exercise is a perfect example of "no pain, no gain." When it is performed correctly, you will feel a burning sensation across the shoulder muscles. If you are not used to working out, do the lowest number of reps until you've gained strength.

**Do 10 reps, increasing to
12 then 15 reps**

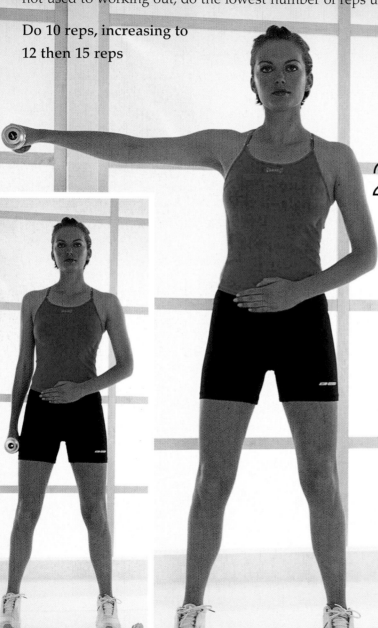

1 Start in a standing position, holding a dumbbell in one hand and the other hand resting on your stomach.

2 Breathe out as you raise the dumbbell to shoulder height. It is of vital importance that the elbows are only slightly bent because this provides the range of motion that directly stresses the posterior deltoid. Inhale as the weight is slowly lowered.

Rest for 2 minutes, then repeat the last 3 exercises before continuing with the program. As you increase the number of reps, rest for 60–90 seconds, then repeat the last 3 exercises 2 to 4 times. Then continue with the program.

gym: workout 4

hammer curl

The hammer curl sculpts and tones the outer sections of the biceps and can actually make your arms appear long, lean, and elegant. Defined biceps help to balance the wider lower half.

Do 20 reps, increasing to 20 reps

1 Stand with feet hip-width apart, legs slightly bent and arms by your sides. Hold the dumbbells so that your palms face inward.

2 Lift the dumbbells toward your shoulders, keeping your elbows tucked in close to your body. Flex your biceps at the top of the movement. Return to the start position. Keep your body strong throughout.

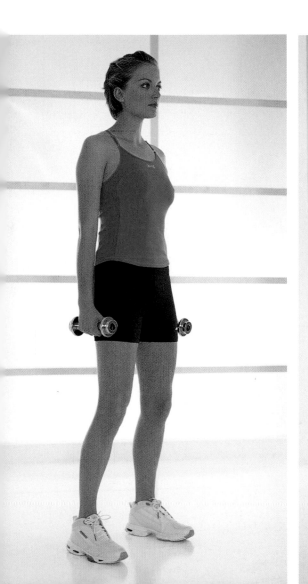

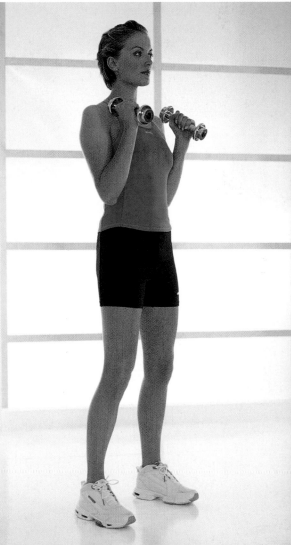

gym: workout 4

triceps kickbacks

This exercise can be done either holding on to the back of a bench (as shown), or standing over a bench with your upper body parallel to the floor. Be sure to keep your arm movements steady, and your arm tight against your side.

Do 10 reps, increasing to 12 then 15 reps

1 Stand with your feet apart. Place your left knee on the bench and left hand against the support. Hold the dumbbell in your right hand, bend your upper body slightly forward. Bring the dumbbell in to your side.

2 Straighten your arm out behind you, then bring it back to your side, gently touching your ribs with the dumbbell.

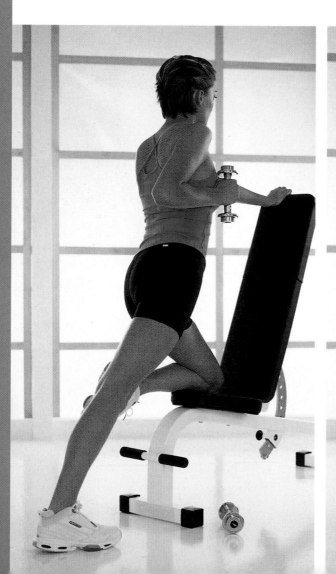

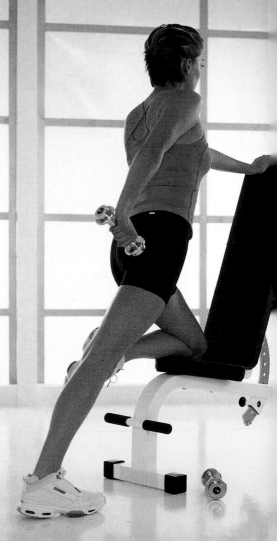

gym: workout 4

straight arm pulldowns

This works the muscles across the back and also the triceps. Use the cable machine with a bar attachment and load the appropriate amount of weight for your fitness level, slowly working your way up to heavier weights as the weeks go by.

Do 12 reps, increasing to 15 then 18 reps

1 Stand facing the cable machine at arm's length away from it, with feet hip-width apart. Grasp the bar in front of you with both hands.

2 Keeping your arms straight, pull the bar down until it reaches your thighs. Hold for 1 second, then return to the start position and repeat.

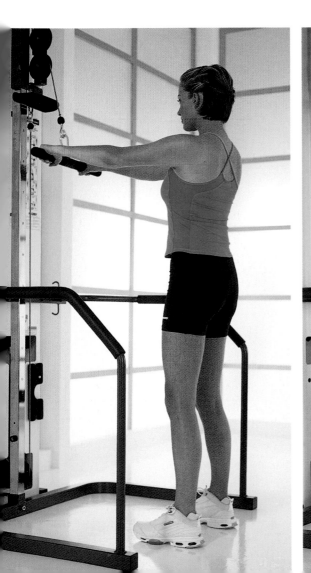

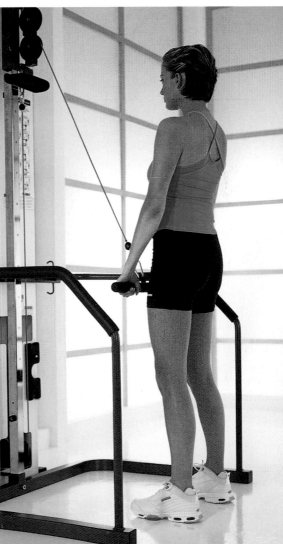

gym: workout 4

cable pull with fitness ball

This exercise can be performed on a cable machine with a platform to help support your weight, or on a pull-up bar. Alternatively, use a fitness ball to sit on, as here. This engages your abdominal muscles, helping to create a strong core for your body.

Do 10 reps, increasing to 15 reps

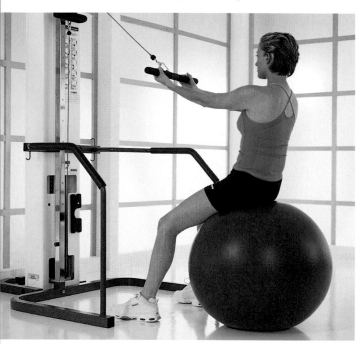

1 Sit on the fitness ball in front of the cable column, about 4–5ft (1.2–1.5m) away from the machine. Gripping your hands underneath the bar, lean back slightly, keeping your feet firmly planted on the ground.

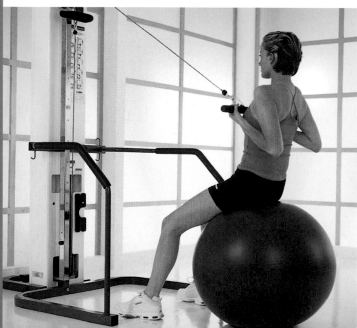

2 Pull the bar back toward your chest, holding your back straight. Return to the start position, keeping your breathing even. Breathe out as you pull the bar toward you, and inhale as you release the bar.

gym: workout 4

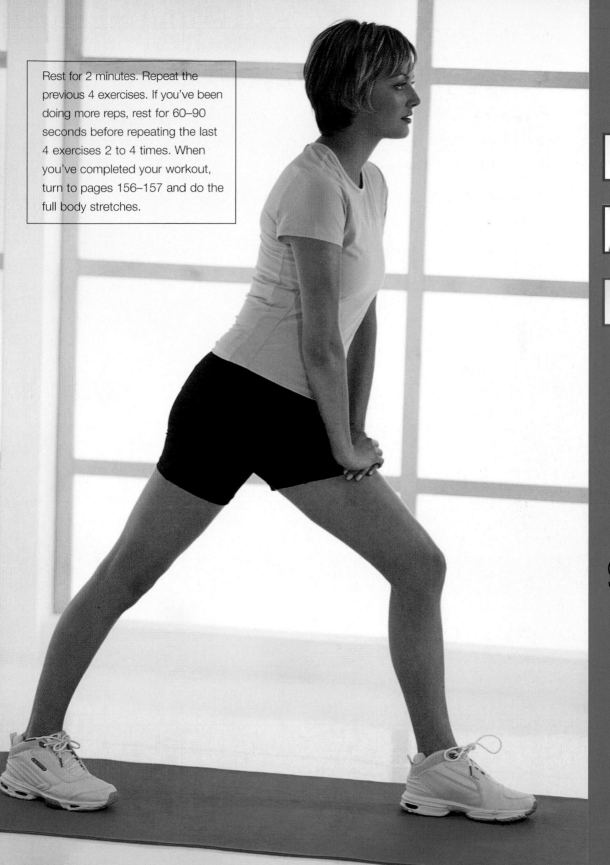

Rest for 2 minutes. Repeat the previous 4 exercises. If you've been doing more reps, rest for 60–90 seconds before repeating the last 4 exercises 2 to 4 times. When you've completed your workout, turn to pages 156–157 and do the full body stretches.

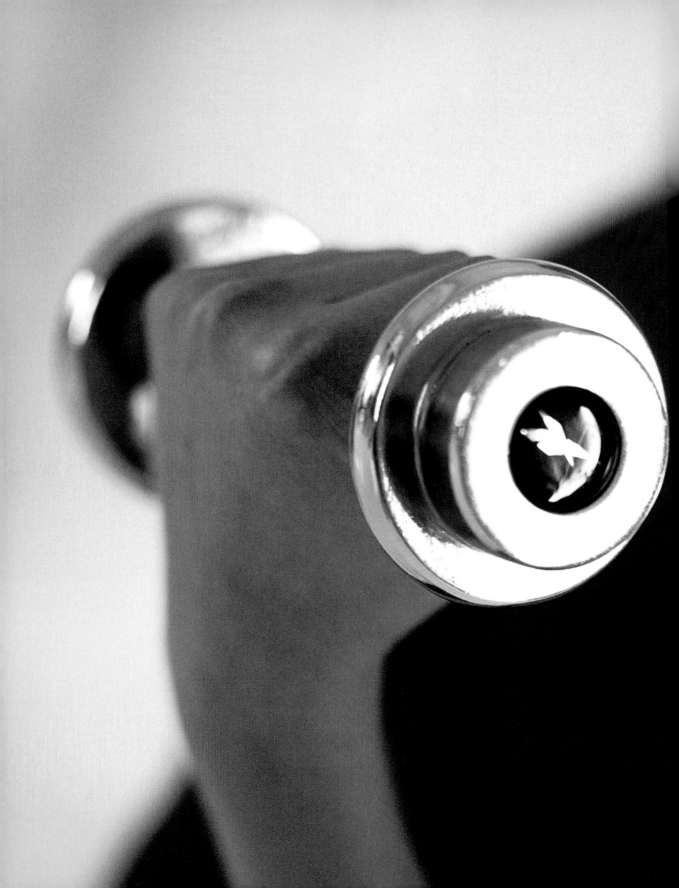

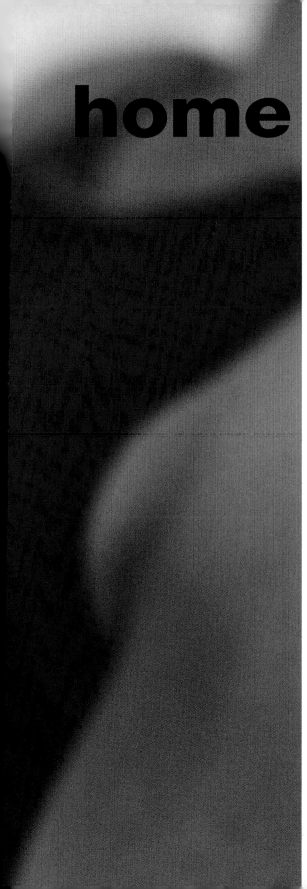

home workouts

In an ideal world, we would go to the gym at least four times a week. But sometimes real life has an irritating way of interfering with plans and sidelining our gym visits. With this in mind, I have created the home workout programs to support your gym visits and ensure that, even if you can't make it out, you can at least benefit from a workout at home. Exercising at home has many advantages. You don't have to travel anywhere, you can do your exercises whenever you choose, and other than a few pieces of equipment, very little outlay is required.

The following workouts can be performed in any home, regardless of space constraints. They can be done on carpet, or on a tiled or hardwood floor. If the floor is not carpeted, it is wise to invest in a nonslip exercise mat or yoga mat, similar to the ones in the photographs. The other pieces of equipment you'll need are a fitness ball, dumbbells, and an exercise tube. Fitness balls are available in three sizes, so choose one according to your height and weight. You can buy any of this equipment from most sports shops and many department stores.

What's preventing you from exercising, once you've assembled your workout equipment and (if necessary) cleared a space? In most cases, it's simply a question of motivation. Because there's no financial investment in working out at home, it may be hard to motivate yourself. Aim to make your exercise routine part of your daily life, first thing in the morning, or as soon as you get home from work. Exercising at regular times helps make your workouts into a habit—one that you won't want to give up when you start to see results.

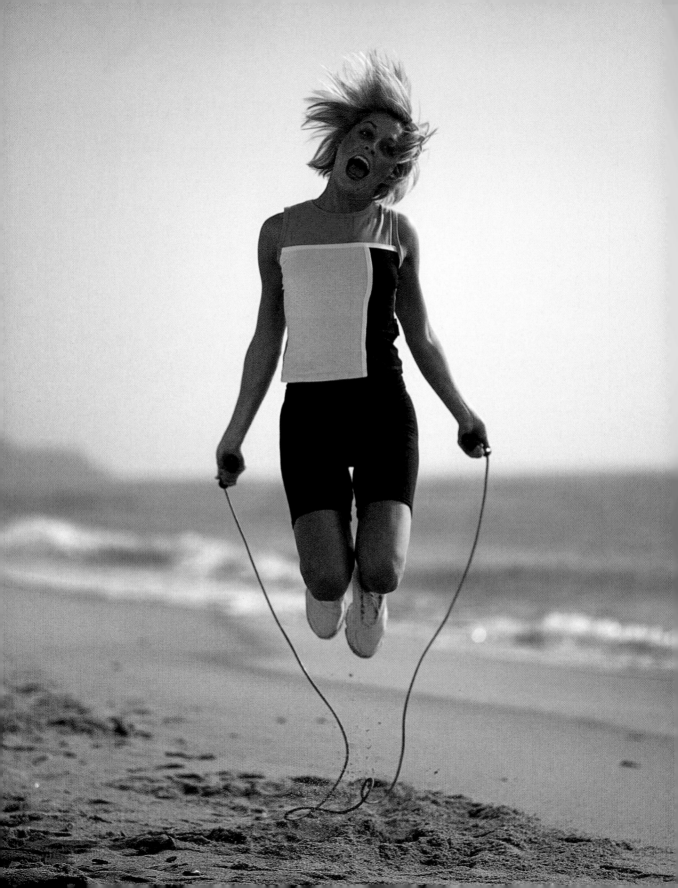

lower body workout 5

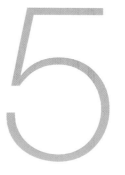

If you dislike the size or shape of your hips, thighs, or buttocks, this workout is designed with you in mind. It works your lower body hard—you'll soon see the difference.

As part of our home training program, we will be focusing on the "problem" areas that typically apply to the apple and hourglass body shapes. That's not to say that tubes and pears shouldn't try this workout—but they should do the program only once through, before turning to the cool-down. Since the hourglass body shape is already well-proportioned, our intention with this workout is to define and tone these curves. The apple body shape, on the other hand, will be making the most of her best asset: long, lean legs. And we'll be adding aerobic exercises, such as jumping rope, to help reduce body fat on the stomach. When doing this workout, move quickly from exercise to exercise unless otherwise stated. Each exercise challenges a different muscle group, allowing the previously worked muscles to rest while maintaining a high workout pace.

home: workout 5

exercise	perform	exercise	perform
jumping rope	50 skips	glute raise	20 reps
ball squat	25 reps	hamstring curl on fitness ball	20 reps
walking lunge	20 lunges	bridge with glute raise	15 reps
fast step-ups	30 steps per leg	bridge	30 secs
basic crunch	20 reps	glute raise on fitness ball	20 reps per side
walking lunge	20 lunges	fitness ball crunch	15 reps
wide leg squat	20 reps	**repeat the workout starting from**	
jump squats	20 reps	**the ball squat**	
fitness ball obliques	20 reps	**cool-down stretches as prescribed**	

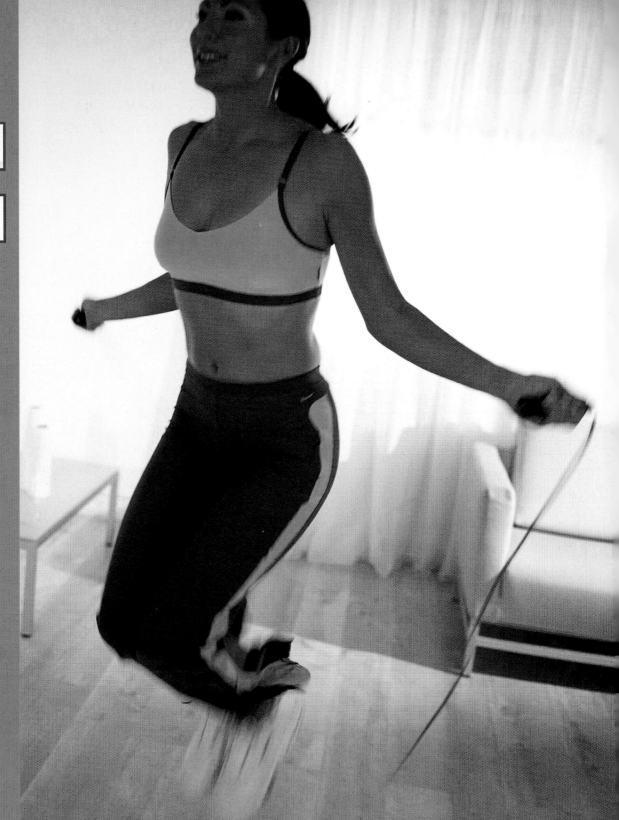

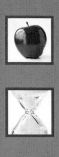

jumping rope

This warm-up is one of my favorite ways to get the heart pumping. After a couple of minutes, your heart will be beating fast and you'll be ready to begin your workout. Best of all, you can do this exercise almost anywhere, anytime.

Do at least 50 jumps

1 Stand with feet together and back straight. Hold the ends of the jump rope in your hands, with the rope behind your heels.

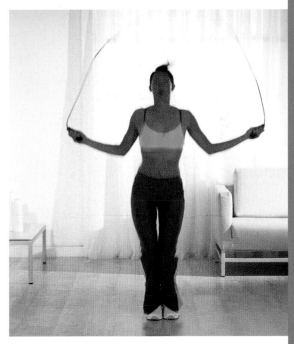

2 Pass the rope over your head and, as it approaches your feet, lightly bounce them off the floor. Aim to keep both feet together and spring from the balls of the feet. Don't jump too high, though, since this can strain your knees. Rest for 30 seconds before moving on.

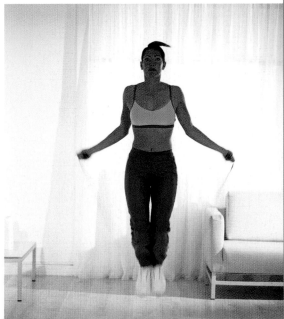

home: warm-up 5

ball squat

Using a fitness ball for this squat allows you to place your body weight farther back toward your heels. This increases the pressure on your inner thighs and buttocks. Keep your neck and shoulders relaxed, and face straight ahead.

Do 25 reps

1 Position the fitness ball between your lower and middle back and a wall. Keep your back straight and arms relaxed by your sides. Your legs should be almost straight.

2 Slowly lower your body until your thighs are parallel to the floor. Then slowly push yourself back up to the starting position, and repeat.

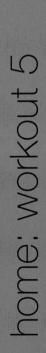

home: workout 5

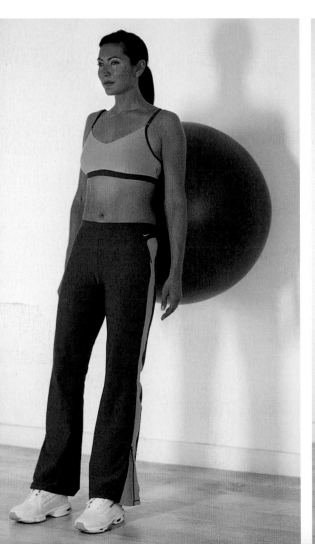

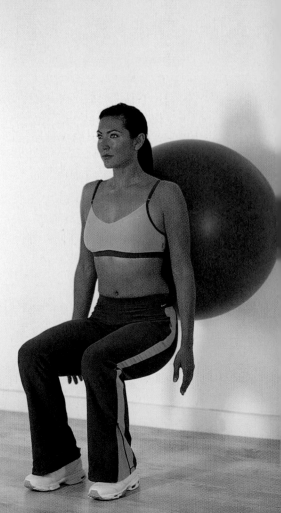

walking lunge

The continuous forward movement of this lunge ensures that all the muscles of the legs and midsection work hard. All four steps are pictured on pages 124–125.

Do 20 lunges

1 Stand with feet hip-width apart and knees slightly bent. Hold the dumbbells by your side.

2 Step forward so that your foot is about one stride-length from your back foot. As you do this, lower your body, then hold the position for 1 second.

3 Raise your body, lifting your back leg as you do so, then, keeping your body straight, move your back foot forward to repeat the lunge with that leg. Use the dumbbells for balance.

4 Step forward another stride-length. Repeat the movement of lowering your body down, and hold again for 1 second. Repeat the required number of lunges, switching direction whenever you need to.

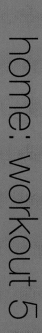

home: workout 5

fast step-ups

You can use stairs or an aerobic step for this move. Just make sure you have enough room to move quickly. The faster you work on the step, the higher your heart rate will get. Result? Your body will burn fat at a faster rate.

Do 30 steps, increasing to 50 steps on each leg

1 Adjust the step so that your knee does not bend to less than 90° when you step onto it.

2 Step up with one foot, placing your foot flat on the step. Keep your back straight and your head and neck relaxed.

3 Step up with your other foot so that both feet are flat on the step. Step down with your leading foot. Repeat, alternating the leading foot.

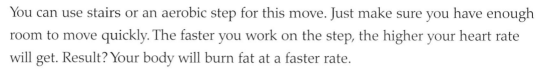

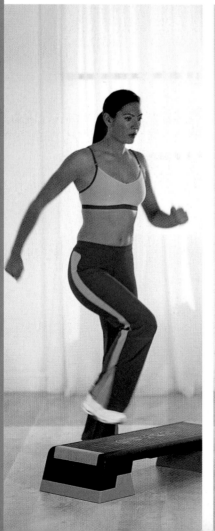

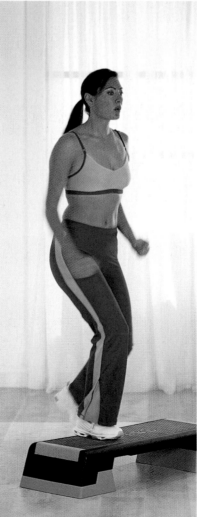

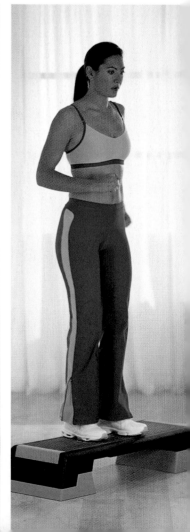

home: workout 5

basic crunch

The basic crunch works the entire stomach area, and is one of the most effective abdominal exercises you can do. Make sure to keep your hips still to get the full benefits of this exercise.

Do 20 reps, increasing to 30 reps

1 Lie on your back with your knees bent, feet flat on the floor and hands by your ears.

2 Curl your shoulders forward, keeping your lower back on the floor. Breathe out as you lift and in as you lower. Keep a space the size of an apple under your chin, to ensure that your head stays in line with your spine. Each repetition should take 4–5 seconds.

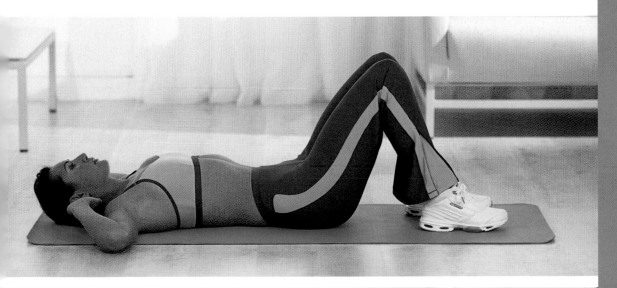

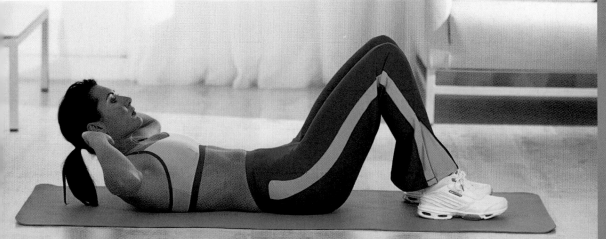

home: workout 5

walking lunge

We repeat this exercise to give your thighs an extra workout. Even though you're probably feeling the strain on your thighs and calf muscles, keep moving. In just a few short weeks of doing this exercise, your legs will be long, lean, and shapely.

Do 20 lunges

1 Stand with feet hip-width apart and knees slightly bent. Hold the dumbbells by your side, palms facing inward.

2 Step forward so that your foot is about one stride-length from your back foot. As you do this, lower your body, then hold the position for 1 second.

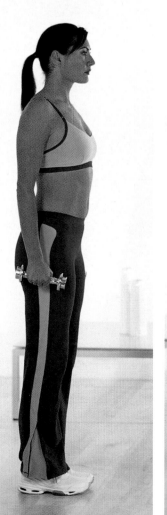

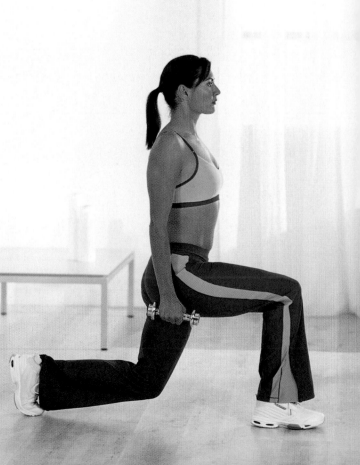

home: workout 5

"After a few reps, your legs may feel weak or wobbly. Persevere with the exercise, though, because the walking lunge is one of the quickest, most effective ways to tone up your backside."

3 Raise your body, lifting your back leg as you do so; then, keeping your body straight, move your back foot forward to repeat the lunge with that leg. Use the dumbbells for balance.

4 Step forward another stride-length. Repeat the movement of lowering your body down, and hold again for 1 second. Repeat the required number of lunges, switching direction whenever you need to.

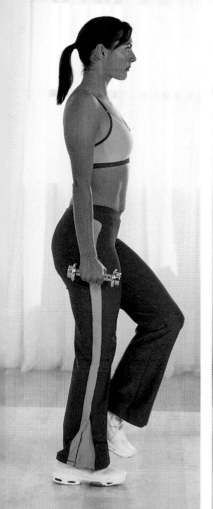

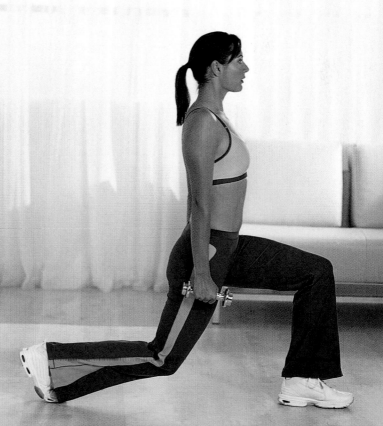

home: workout 5

wide leg squat

This is an excellent move to help tone up the rear end and inner thighs. It's important to keep your knees facing outward at all times. To achieve quicker results, tighten your buttocks before starting. The dumbbell makes it harder.

Do 20 reps

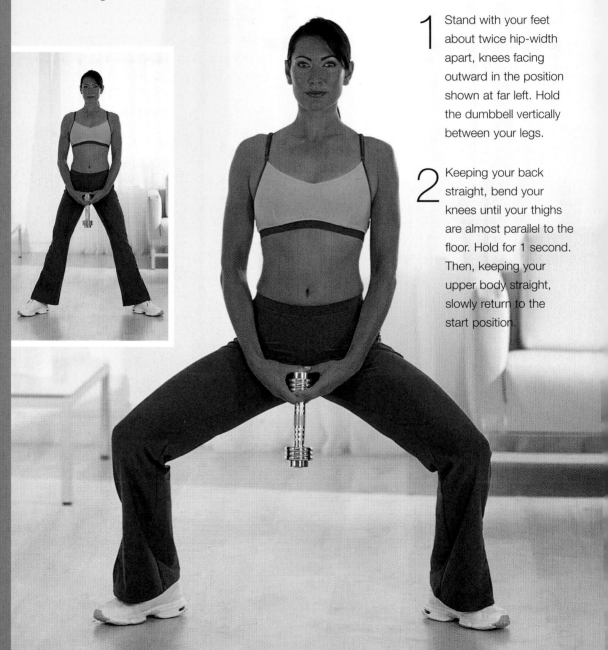

1 Stand with your feet about twice hip-width apart, knees facing outward in the position shown at far left. Hold the dumbbell vertically between your legs.

2 Keeping your back straight, bend your knees until your thighs are almost parallel to the floor. Hold for 1 second. Then, keeping your upper body straight, slowly return to the start position.

home: workout 5

jump squats

Using a medicine ball with this exercise increases the intensity of your workout. Keep your eyes fixed on a point in front of you so that you don't lose your balance. Do the exercise slowly to avoid placing strain on your knee joints.

Do 20 reps

1 Starting in the crouch position, hold the medicine ball at chest height, as if to do an overhand throw. Keep your elbows soft, and your neck and shoulders relaxed.

2 Inhale and spring up, keeping the ball steady at chest height. Your legs should be straight and strong. Land toes first, and return to the crouch position. Repeat.

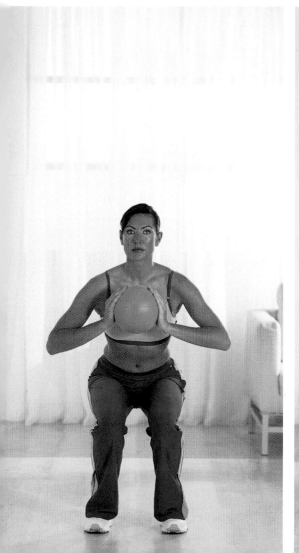

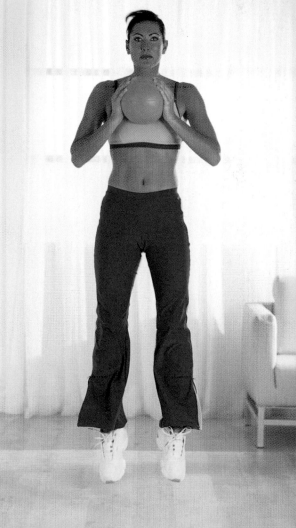

home: workout 5

fitness ball obliques

Resting your legs on the fitness ball in this exercise makes you work your waist muscles harder as you rotate your body. Make sure you are steady before beginning this exercise—use your legs as stabilizers.

Do 20 reps on each side

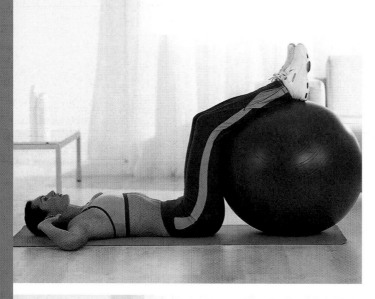

1 Lie flat on your back, with your heels and calves resting close together on the fitness ball. Make sure you tuck the fitness ball in tight against your thighs. Place your hands by your ears.

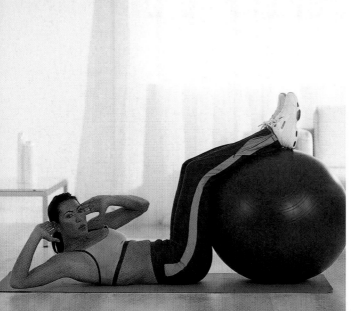

2 Slowly raise one shoulder and one elbow toward your opposite knee. Slowly return to the start. Lift your other shoulder and elbow for the next raise, then continue alternating sides until you've completed all the reps.

home: workout 5

glute raise

This tones the muscles in your buttocks (glutes) to lift you
firmer, more pert appearance. To maximize the lifting effec
and hold your tummy muscles tight. Keep your hips flat o

Do 20 reps, increasing to 30 reps, on each leg

1 Lie on your front, with your forehead
resting on your hands. Raise one leg
so your knee forms a right angle.

2 Squeeze yo
of your foot
possible. L
all your reps, then switch legs and repeat.

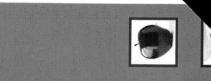

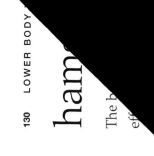

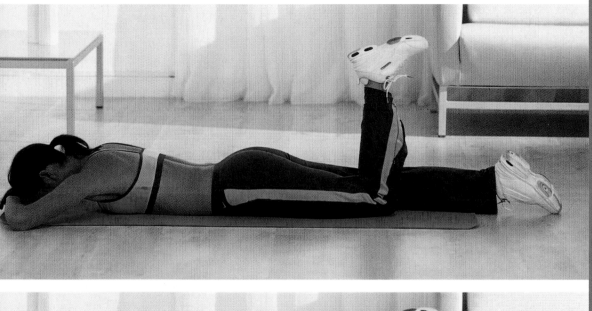

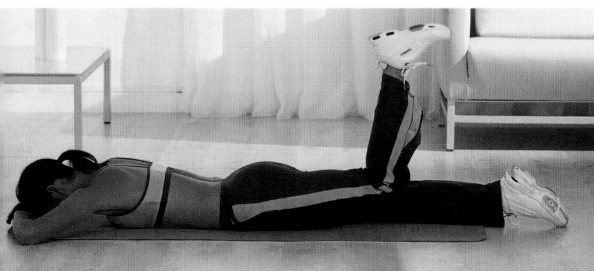

string curl on fitness ball

est non-gym exercise for the backs of your thighs. To make it even more
ective, raise your hips off the floor in step one and then keep them raised.
Use your arms to steady yourself.

Do 20 reps, increasing to 30 reps

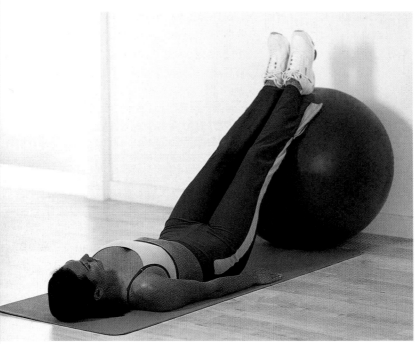

1 Place the fitness ball against a wall. Lie on your back with your arms by your sides and your palms on the floor. Rest your feet on the middle of the ball. Keep your heels knee-width apart and your toes pointing up. To get the most out of this exercise, remember to keep the hips raised off the floor at all times.

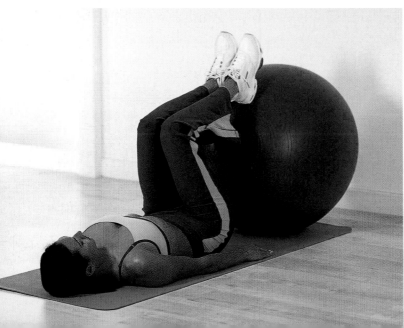

2 Gently push your heels into the top of the ball, then pull them slowly toward you, dragging the ball about 8in (20cm) toward you as you do so. Keep your head, shoulders, and arms still. Slowly return your legs and the fitness ball to the start position.

home: workout 5

bridge with glute raise

This is a great waist-whittler—as long as you do it correctly. Keep yourself steady by squeezing your stomach muscles tight. Begin with small 6in (15cm) leg lifts, working your way up to higher 12in (30cm) lifts as you get stronger.

Do 15 reps, increasing to 25 reps, on each side

1 Position yourself with your toes on the floor and your elbows and forearms directly under your shoulders. Raise yourself up so you're supporting your body with your elbows, forearms, and toes.

2 Raise one leg 6in (15cm). Hold for 20–40 seconds, keeping your body as still and strong as possible. Return to the start. Complete all the reps on one side, then switch legs and repeat.

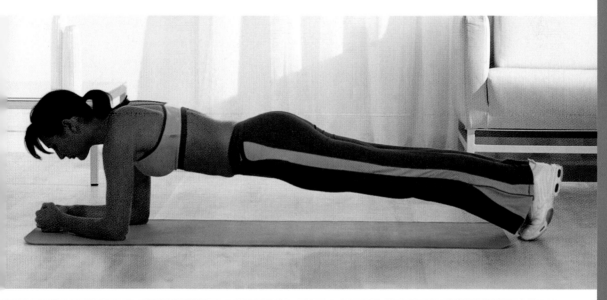

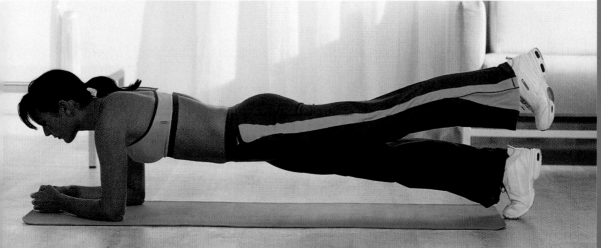

home: workout 5

bridge

This is a static exercise that helps to strengthen the muscles in the stomach and lower back. It is an advanced exercise and should be attempted only by stronger exercisers, so work your way up slowly.

Hold for 30 seconds, increasing to 60 seconds

1 Position yourself so that your toes are on the ground and your elbows are directly below your shoulders. Raise yourself up, keeping a straight line from your shoulders.

2 Use your abdominals to maintain the position. Be careful not to stick your backside up in the air. Hold for 30 seconds.

home: workout 5

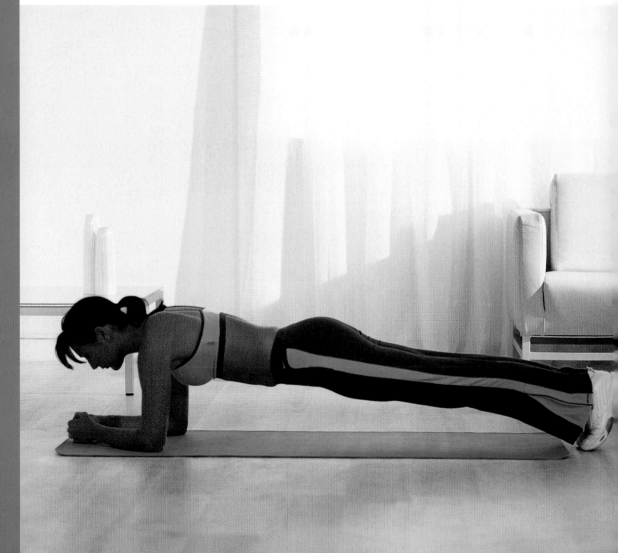

glute raise on fitness ball

This exercise calls for strength and stability to keep your balance. Here's where your stomach muscles count, so it's important to keep them as strong and firm as possible. Don't tense your shoulders—your fingers should lightly touch the ground.

Do 20 reps, increasing to 30 reps, on each side

1 Lie across a fitness ball, stretching your arms out in front of you to provide balance. Stretch your legs out as far as they will go behind you, keeping your toes on the ground.

2 Keeping your stomach muscles firm, raise one leg about 8in (20cm) off the ground. Hold for 1 second before lowering. Repeat. Once you've completed your reps on one leg, switch to the other leg.

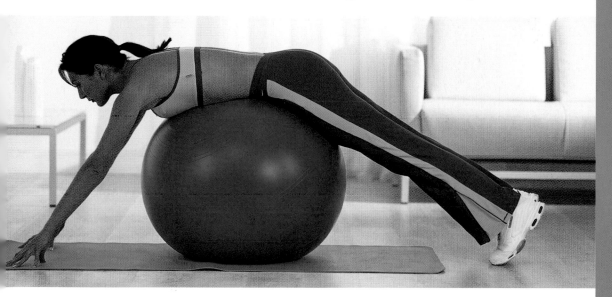

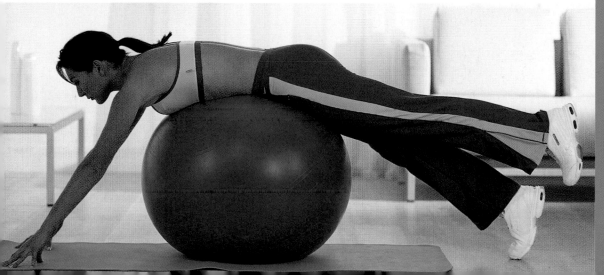

home: workout 5

fitness ball crunch

If you really want to work your stomach muscles, then this is the perfect exercise for you. By using those muscles to control your balance, you'll be giving them an even harder and more effective workout.

Do 15 reps, increasing to 30 reps

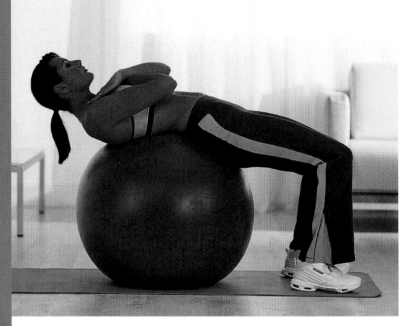

1 Sit on the fitness ball, with your feet firmly in front of you. Taking small steps, move your legs forward so that your body begins to move down the ball. Stop once the ball reaches the middle of your back. Cross your arms over your chest. Tighten your stomach muscles to prepare for step 2.

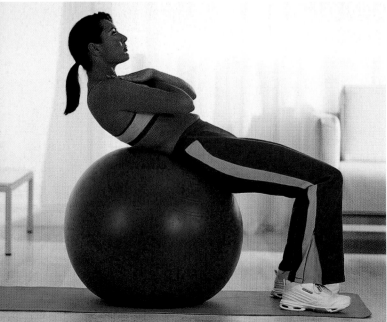

2 Inhaling, raise your upper body halfway off the ball, or until you can feel a distinct tightening in your stomach muscles. Lower to the start position in a smooth and controlled movement, and repeat.

home: workout 5

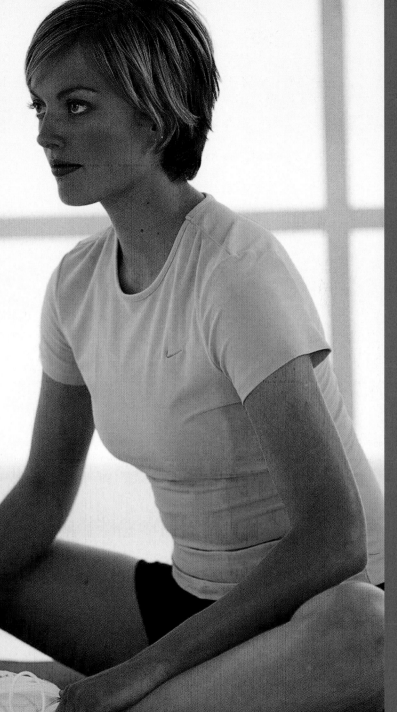

What next?
Repeat the sequence of exercises, minus the rope-jumping warm-up. Then turn to page 157 and complete the lower body stretch (the inner thigh stretch is shown here).

Moving forward
• As you get stronger, you can repeat this program three times.

• Use dumbbells in the ball squat (page 120) to make the exercise more intense.

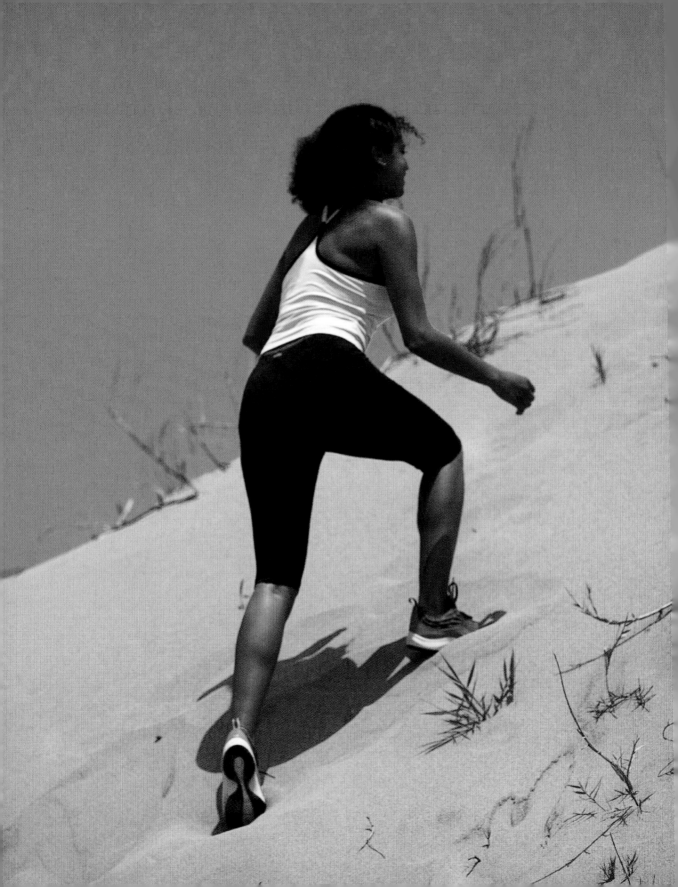

total body workout 6

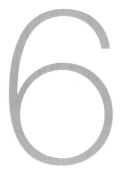

This program is designed as a complete all-arounder, providing a great home workout, helping you achieve a leaner, more toned figure—no matter what your body shape.

Exercising at home does not need to be any less effective than time spent at the gym. The secret is to choose the right type of exercises for your environment. This workout is broken into sections, which isolate and intensively work specific body parts before moving on to a brief "aerobic" blitz. These additions are designed to raise your body's temperature significantly and increase its potential to burn fat effectively. The isolated exercises produce an enormous amount of "muscle utilization" from each area that is being worked, providing significant gains in your body's efficiency and performance capability. The program works each area just hard enough to achieve visible changes without increasing body mass.

home: workout 6

exercise	perform	exercise	perform
jogging in place	5 min	biceps curls	30 reps
squats	20 reps	jumping rope	30 secs
body lift	20 reps	ab crunches	20 reps
power lunge	20 reps	oblique crosses (alternate)	30 reps
donkey kicks	15 reps	back extension	20 reps
jogging in place	30 secs	reverse curl	15 reps
triceps dips	15 reps	step-ups	30 reps
shoulder press	20 reps per side	**repeat all exercises except the warm-up**	
lateral raises	15 reps	**cool-down stretches as prescribed**	

jogging in place

If you can't go for a run outside, you can jog in place and receive the same warm-up benefits.

Do 5 minutes

1 Standing with your feet hip-width apart, lift your leg as though you were going to take a short step forward. Quickly lower it, bouncing from one foot to the other.

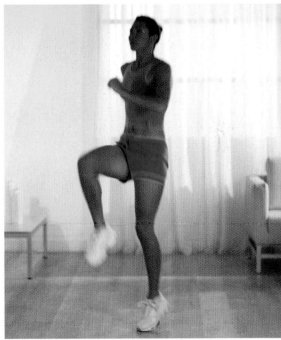

2 Repeat until you have completed the warm-up time. Take short, fast steps, and don't bring your knees up too high. Keep your arms loosely bent, and face forward with your neck and shoulders relaxed and your back straight and strong.

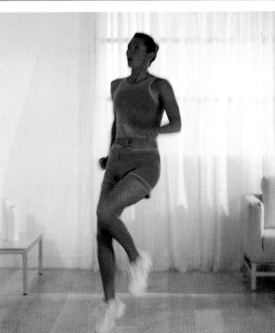

home: warm-up 6

squats

This exercise will help to get your heart rate going and warm up the lower body muscle groups. Take care to keep your stomach pulled in tight and your rear end tucked under.

Do 20 reps, increasing to 25, then 30 reps

1 Stand with your feet hip-width apart and knees slightly bent. Keep your back straight and your hands on your hips.

2 Bend your knees to about 90°, allowing your body to lean forward slightly until it is at right angles to your thighs. Keep your feet still. Return to the start and repeat.

home: workout 6

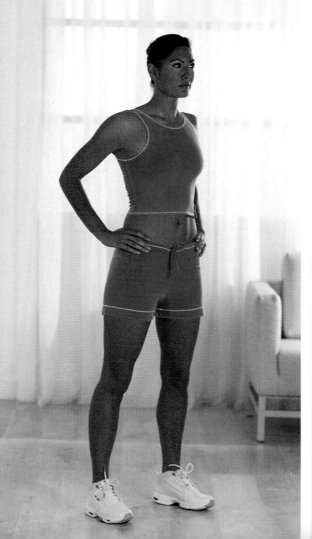
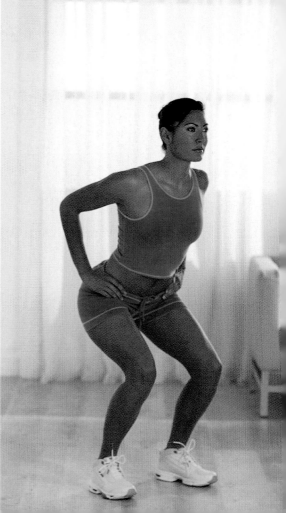

body lift

This is an intensive workout for your rear end and the backs of your legs. If you're a beginner or out of shape, then point your toes upward; otherwise, make the move harder by pointing your toes away from you.

Do 20 reps, increasing to 30 reps

1 Lie on your back with your heels on a step or low chair, and your knees at 90°. Place your arms by your sides, palms facing down.

2 Raise your pelvis until your body is straight from your knees to your chest. Pointing your toes up or away from you, squeeze your buttocks. Slowly lower to the start position. Repeat.

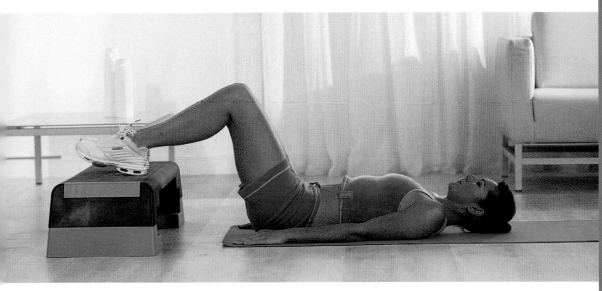

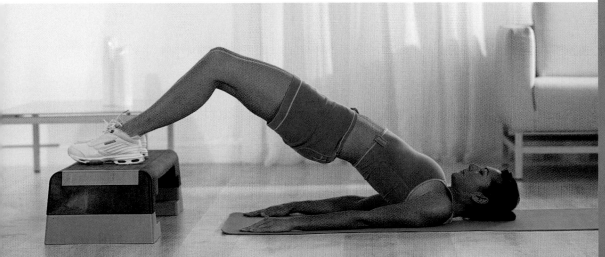

home: workout 6

power lunge

A demanding exercise, this lunge works the muscles in the legs and hips and can give you wonderfully toned inner thighs and buttocks. For best results, take it slowly: two or three seconds on the way down and the same on the way up.

Do 20 reps, increasing to 30 reps, then 40 reps with practice

1 Stand with feet hip-width apart, and hands on your hips. Face straight ahead and place one foot forward about one stride-length from the back leg.

2 Bend your knees to bring your front knee directly over your front foot. The movement should be downward rather than forward; put your weight onto the heel of your front foot to work the buttock muscle most effectively. Return to the start; repeat.

home: workout 6

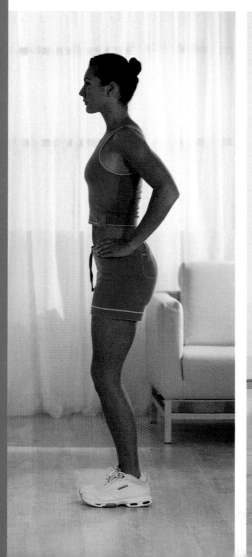

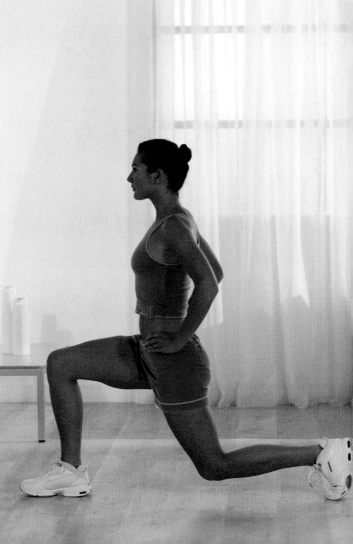

donkey kicks

This is a fantastic exercise to help tone the inner thighs. This area is quite difficult to sculpt and strengthen and is often neglected during a workout. Within a couple of weeks, you should also notice a lifting and firmness of your rear end.

Do 15 reps on each side, increasing to 25 reps, then 30 reps with practice

1 Kneel on all fours, resting on your hands, elbows, and forearms. Keep your head facing down and point your toes.

2 Kick one leg directly back, so that your body is at an angle. Return to the start position. Complete all the reps on one side, then do the other.

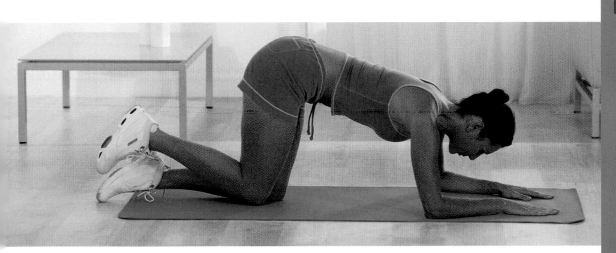

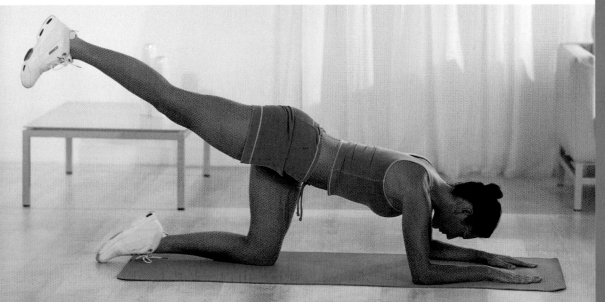

home: workout 6

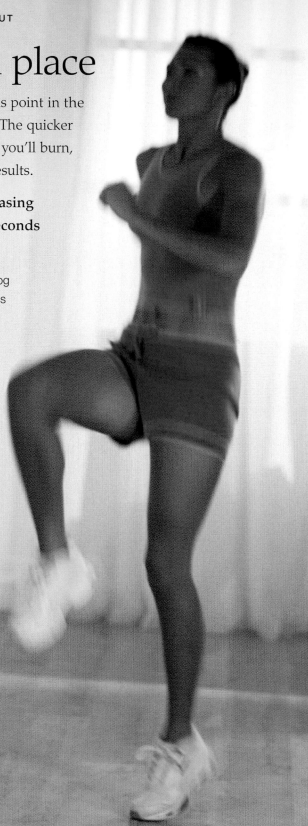

jogging in place

Revitalize your body at this point in the workout with a quick jog. The quicker you jog, the more calories you'll burn, and the faster you'll see results.

Jog for 30 seconds, increasing to 45 seconds, then 60 seconds

Speed up your heart rate and jog quickly in place. Keep your arms loose and your tread firm.

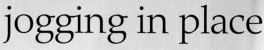

home: workout 6

triceps dips

This is a exceptionally good way to define and strengthen the triceps. You can make it more difficult by moving your feet as far away as possible from the support.

Do 15 reps, increasing to 20 reps, then 25 reps with practice

1 Standing with your back to a sofa or bench, position your heels 2–3ft (60–90cm) in front of you. Grip the edge of the support with an overhand wide grip (palms down) and push yourself up so that your arms are fully extended and perpendicular to the floor.

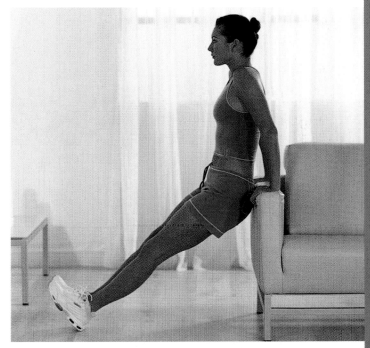

2 Bending your arms, descend toward the floor until your upper arms are parallel to the floor. Push back up to the starting position. Repeat.

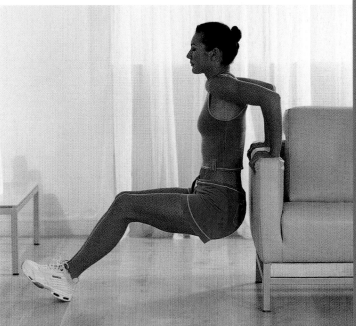

home: workout 6

shoulder press

This exercise works the deltoids, or shoulder muscles. Make sure you have enough of the exercise tube under your feet to hold it firm.

Do 20 reps each side, increasing to 30 reps, then 40 reps with practice

1 Grasp the exercise tube behind your arm so that your elbow is bent at 90°. Keep your abdominals tight at all times.

2 Lift your arm straight up. Exhale as you extend and take care not to lock your arm straight. Breathe in as you return to the start position.

home: workout 6

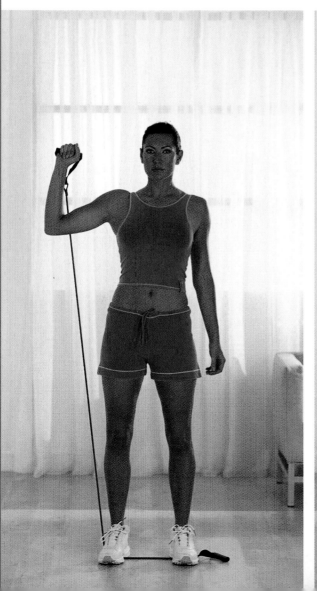
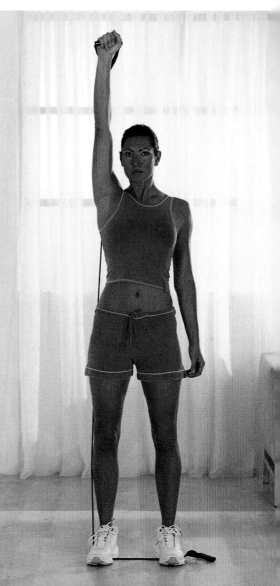

lateral raises

This exercise also works the deltoids. In step two, keep your torso still to ensure that you work all three sections of the shoulder muscles.

**Do 15 reps, increasing to
20 reps, then 25 reps
with practice**

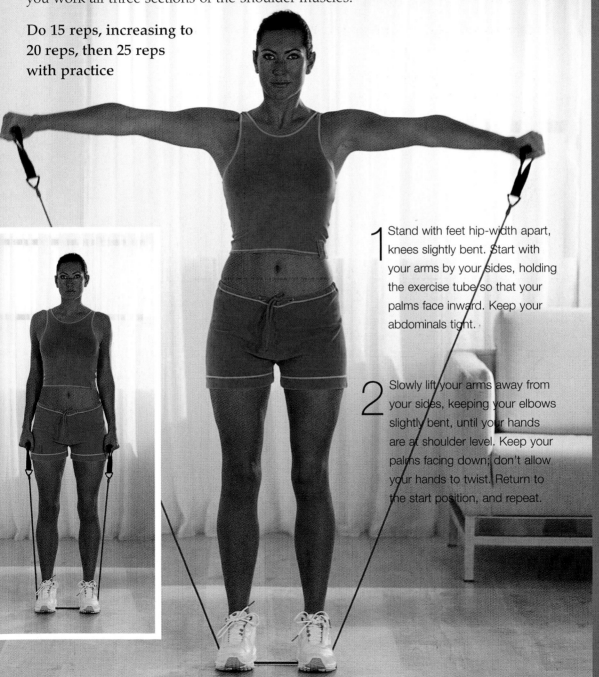

1 Stand with feet hip-width apart, knees slightly bent. Start with your arms by your sides, holding the exercise tube so that your palms face inward. Keep your abdominals tight.

2 Slowly lift your arms away from your sides, keeping your elbows slightly bent, until your hands are at shoulder level. Keep your palms facing down; don't allow your hands to twist. Return to the start position, and repeat.

home: workout 6

biceps curls (alternating)

This is an exceptionally good and intensive exercise for all body shapes, since it creates definition and strength in the biceps.

Do 30 reps, increasing to 40 reps, then 50 reps with practice

1 Stand on the exercise tube with feet hip-width apart. Gripping the handles of the tube, bend your right arm toward your shoulder, keeping the left arm by your side.

2 Lower your right arm, then lift the left arm toward your shoulder. Keep your body strong and the movement slow and controlled as you complete the reps, alternating arms.

home: workout 6

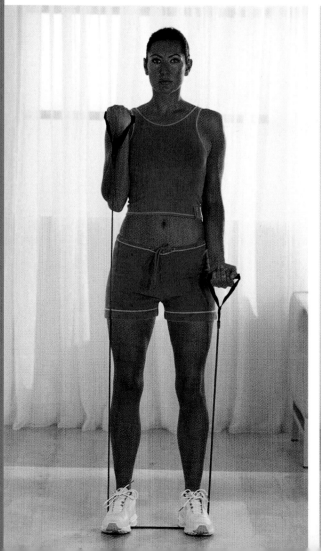

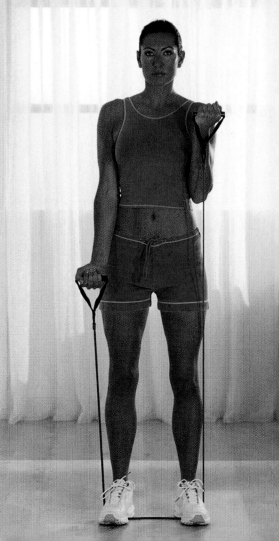

jumping rope

This is one of the quickest ways to raise your heart rate. Jumping rope tones your entire body and requires very little time and effort. Begin slowly, working your way up to the more advanced level.

Do 30 seconds, increasing to 45 seconds, then 60 seconds with practice

Stand with feet together and back straight. Hold the ends of the jump rope in your hands, with the rope behind your heels. Pass the rope over your head and, as it approaches your feet, lightly bounce them off the floor. Aim to keep both feet together and spring from the balls of the feet. Don't jump too high, since this can jar your knees. Rest for 30 seconds before moving on to the next exercise.

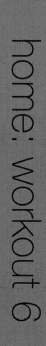

home: workout 6

ab crunches

An extremely effective abdominal exercise. Keep the movement slow and controlled, concentrating on good technique, and your eyes focused on the ceiling.

Do 20 reps, increasing to 40 reps, then 50 reps with practice

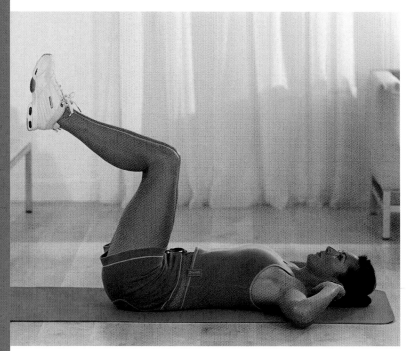

1 Lie on your back with your legs in the air, knees bent, and your hands by your ears.

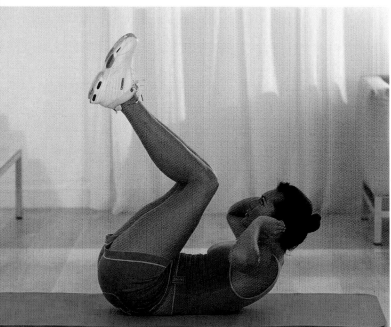

2 Curl your legs and pelvis toward your rib cage. At the same time, curl your shoulders forward, keeping your lower back on the floor. Tense the abdominals, breathing out as you lift and in as you lower slowly to the start position. Each repetition should take about 4–5 seconds.

home: workout 6

oblique crosses (alternate)

Raising your legs in the air for this exercise means you use your abdominal muscles to keep your balance. Keep your legs together to maximize the effort.

Do 30 reps, increasing to 40 reps, then 50 reps with practice

1 Lie on your back with your knees together and legs raised so that your thighs are at 90° to the floor. Keep your tummy muscles pulled in tight and your back pressed into the floor. Place your hands by your ears.

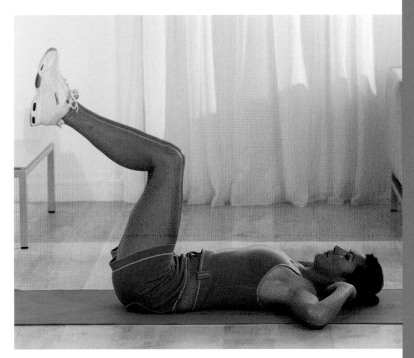

2 Raise one elbow and shoulder toward your opposite knee. Return to the start. Do the next oblique with your other elbow, and then alternate sides until you've completed all the reps.

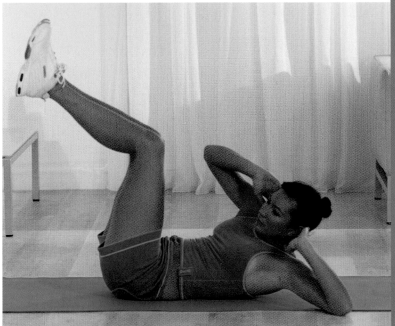

home: workout 6

back extension

This exercise concentrates on strengthening your back. It improves your posture and is a particularly good exercise to do if you spend a lot of time sitting down.

Do 20 reps, increasing to 30 reps, then 40 reps with practice

1 Lie down flat on your front on the floor. Place your hands on either side of your head, keeping your head down.

2 Breathe out and at the same time raise your head and upper body off the floor, taking care not to tense the neck muscles. Hold for 1 second, then breathe in as you lower yourself to the floor. Maintain a slow and controlled movement at all times.

home: workout 6

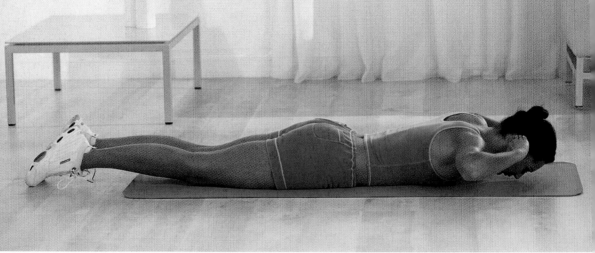

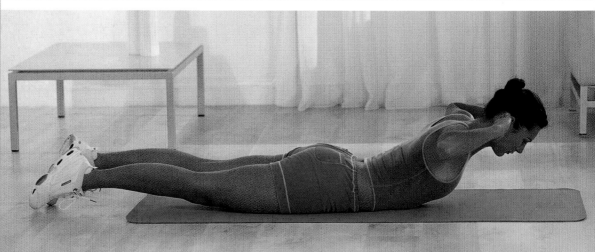

reverse curl

A nice complement to the back extension shown opposite, this exercise helps to strengthen and tone the abdomen from the lower part up.

Do 15 reps, increasing to 25 reps, then 30 reps with practice

1 Lie on your back with your arms out to the sides, legs in the air. Keep your shoulders and head on the floor at all times.

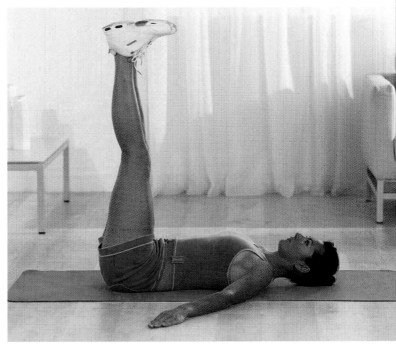

2 Tighten your lower abdominals and curl your legs and pelvis toward your rib cage. Make sure your feet never come back farther than your head. Hold for 1 second, then return to the start position, using your stomach muscles to control the movement.

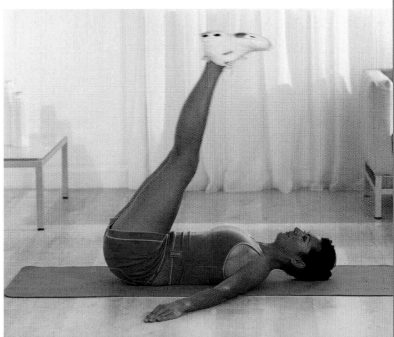

home: workout 6

step-ups

Work briskly through this exercise. Step-ups work your lower body muscles, but they should also raise your heart rate. If you don't have an exercise step, use the stairs. Just make sure that the step isn't too high—you shouldn't be lifting your knees higher than your hips.

Do 30 reps, increasing to 45 reps, then 60 reps with practice

Stand facing a step or stair. Step up with one foot, placing your whole foot flat on the step. Keep your back straight and your head and neck relaxed but in line with your torso. Step up with your other foot so that both feet are flat on the step. Step down one foot at a time. Repeat until you've done all the reps.

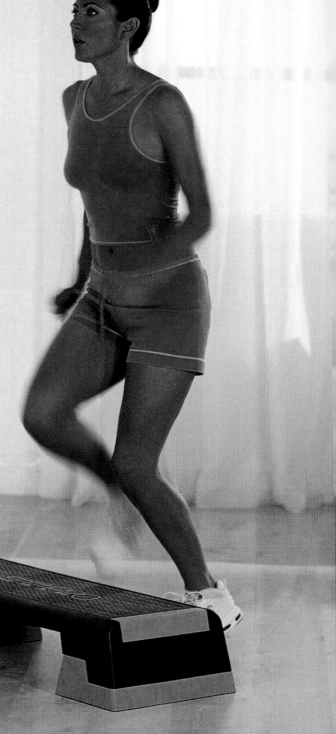

home: workout 6

What next?

Repeat this sequence starting from the squats (page 140). Once you've done all the exercises again, turn to pages 156–157 and do the full body stretch (the triceps stretch is shown here).

Moving forward

• Good technique is important, so concentrate on improving it.

• Aim to increase your workout to the maximum number of reps within four weeks of beginning the program.

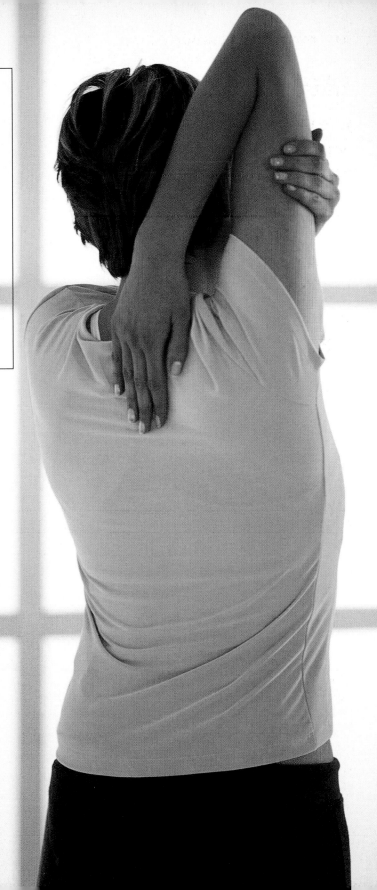

upper body stretch

cool-down stretches

Upper back stretch With your feet hip-width apart and legs slightly bent, straighten your arms out in front, hands clasped. Push your hands away from you to feel the stretch. Hold for 15 seconds.

Triceps stretch Stand as before. Raise one arm and place the hand over your back. Gently push the elbow back with your other hand. Hold for 10 seconds, then repeat the stretch with the other arm.

Chest stretch Stand as before. Clasp your hands behind your back. Lift your arms behind you until you can feel the stretch across your chest. Hold for 15 seconds, then return to the start.

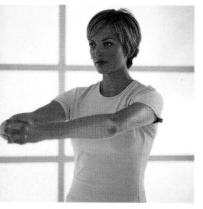

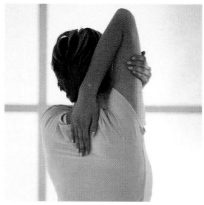

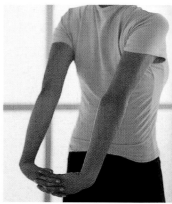

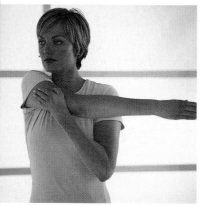

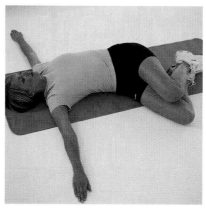

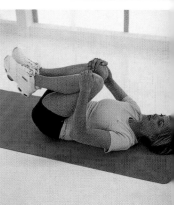

Shoulder stretch Stand as before. Bend your right arm across your body so your forearm is by your left shoulder. Place your left hand on your upper arm to stretch a bit farther. Hold for 10 seconds, then repeat with the other arm.

Spine rotation Lie on your back, arms outstretched. Bend both legs to 90°, then drop your knees to one side so one knee touches the floor. Keep your shoulders flat on the floor. Hold for 15 seconds, then repeat on the other side.

Lower back Lie on your back. Holding the tops of your shins, bring both knees in close to your chest until you can feel the stretch in your lower back. Hold for 10 seconds, then slowly return to the start position.

lower body stretch

Glute stretch Lie on your back, right knee bent and right foot on the floor. Cross your left leg over. Holding behind the right thigh, pull your leg toward you. Hold for 10 seconds. Repeat with the left leg.

Hamstring stretch Place your right foot on a step and straighten your right leg. Bend your left leg slightly. Bend from the hips until you feel the stretch, then hold for 8 seconds. Repeat with the left leg.

Calf stretch Stand feet together. Step back with one foot, pushing into the heel and bending your other leg slightly. Keep your heels on the floor. Hold for 8 seconds. Repeat with the other leg.

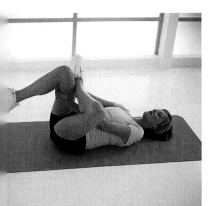
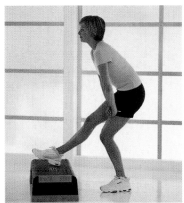
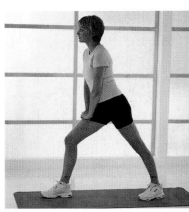

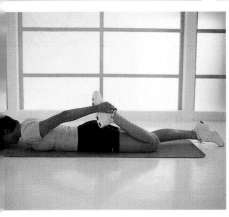
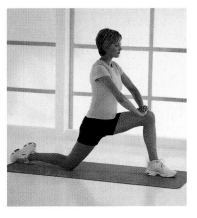
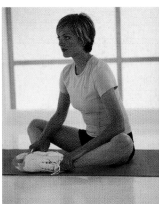

Prone quadriceps stretch Lie face down on the floor. Bring one leg up behind you to hold the foot. Keep your hips on the floor and head down. Hold for 10 seconds. Repeat with the other leg.

Hip flexor Kneel down, then step forward with one foot. Slide your back leg behind you. Straighten up and place both hands on your front knee. Hold for 10 seconds. Repeat with the other leg.

Inner thigh stretch Sit with your back straight. Place the soles of your feet together. Holding your ankles, pull your feet in toward you. Hold for 10 seconds, then gently ease the stretch a little farther.

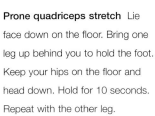

cool-down stretches

exercises by body shape

about the author

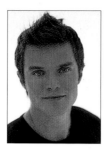

Matt Roberts, the UK's hottest personal trainer, began his career in fitness as an international sprinter. He went on to complete his studies at the American Council for Exercise and the American College of Sports Medicine. Known as "the personal trainer to the stars," Matt has a worldwide reputation for training celebrities, including Sandra Bullock, Trudie Styler, Mel C, Natalie Imbruglia, Naomi Campbell, Tom Ford, John Galliano, and Faye Dunaway. Alongside his work with high-profile clients, he gets equal satisfaction from helping each person he trains to meet his or her health and fitness goals. And in his quest to make wellness accessible to everyone, he produces his own range of vitamins, home gym equipment, and body care products.

author's credits

As always, there are many people I have to thank in helping me put my vision into reality. Firstly, I must thank the wonderful team at DK: Mary-Clare, Gillian, and Karen, who have all worked on developing the book. I would like to also thank Charmaine, my editor, and Bev and Nigel, my brilliant design team. As always, my brother Jon has been a tower of strength and support, not only in the writing of this book, but with the everyday details. And of course nothing would be possible without the love and support of my wife Helen and my daughter Amber.
For more information, please contact:
matt roberts personal training, 32–34 Jermyn Street, London SW1Y 6HS, UK
Telephone +44 (0)20 7439 8800; www.personaltrainer.uk.com

publisher's credits

Many items were kindly loaned for the book. Special thanks to the UK distributor of Cybex (www.cybexintl.com) for equipment used in the gym photographs; Reebok (www.reebok.com) for clothing and shoes; sweatyBetty (www.sweatybetty.com) for their wonderful range of fitness gear; Donna Karan Intimates for their underwear range (available from better department stores). Thanks also to models Elizabeth Howells and Lucy Shakespeare at ModelPlan; Louise Cole, Christianne Gadd, Melanie Liburd, and Carol Rorich at MOT; and to Stephen McIlmoyle and Julie McGuire for hair and makeup.